Shelley Nathans' new volume, *More About Couples on the Couch*, is a wonderful collection of clinical and theoretical articles. International contributions are drawn from leading members of Tavistock Relationships in London, the faculty of the Psychoanalytic Couple Psychotherapy Group in the San Francisco Bay Area, along with other leading therapists who illuminate areas of couple relationships that have been largely out of the spotlight: creativity and imagination, love as a creative illusion, no-sex couples, and same-sex couples, along with a variety of psychoanalytic theoretical contributions. This volume offers a treasure trove the well-read couple therapist will not want to miss.

**David Scharff**,
*co-founder and former director,
International Psychotherapy Institute and former chair,
the International Psychoanalytic Association's Committee
on Couple and Family Psychoanalysis*

In this second volume of *Couples on the Couch*, the seminal book on psychoanalytic couple psychotherapy, we see the merit and value of expansions in theory that allow new ideas and therapeutic projects to emerge. Most importantly, how deeply resonant these innovations are for couples where issues of culture, race, identity, and sexuality are central. This excellent edited volume of papers by international scholars will help therapists understand and work with different kinds of relational configurations and the complex process of undoing, divorcing, or repairing the damages and strains in contemporary relationships.

**Adrienne Harris**,
*New York University Postdoctoral Program in
Psychoanalysis and Psychotherapy*

In this second collection of papers under the title of *Couples on the Couch*, Shelley Nathans has brought together papers from a variety of theoretical orientations, complementing her first collection (co-edited with Milton Schaefer), which took a primarily contemporary Kleinian object relations approach, developed at Tavistock Relationships in London, in its theoretical understanding of human growth and development.

In this collection, Nathans includes an impressive array of papers using the writings of Winnicott, Bollas, Ogden, Fairbairn and Kohut, and the theoretical orientations offered by field, mentalisation, relational and link theories, and by Self Psychology. Each paper is followed by a discussion, which is very often as substantial as the paper to which it is

responding, and together they offer complementary, supplementary, and sometimes alternative emphases on in-depth psychoanalytic work with couples.

Though the Tavistock Relationships model has roots in Jungian (Alison Lyons, Janet Mattinson) and Independent tradition (Enid Balint, Michael Balint) thinking, its subsequent development leaned heavily on the Kleinian and post-Kleinian object relations understanding of the processes of splitting, projective identification, narcissism, and containment as being fundamental to an in-depth exploration of the psychic structure of intimate couple relating. These remain as cornerstones, but the papers in this collection demonstrate how further theoretical constructs substantially add to and develop this understanding.

Using many clinical vignettes all the papers demonstrate how the orientation which they discuss is applied to the clinical work with couples in the consulting room.

What this volume demonstrates, as did the first, is the efficacy of psychoanalytic understanding and treatment in the therapeutic work with intimate couple relationships, and not just with individuals which is where these theories were first developed. More than that, again, as with the first volume, these papers implicitly demonstrate how an understanding of the intrapersonal and interpersonal dynamics of intimate couple interaction informs and strengthens our theories about and clinical practice with individuals.

**Stanley Ruszczynski**,
*psychoanalyst, BPA (British Psychoanalytic Association),*
*IPA, and psychoanalytic couple psychotherapist*

# More About Couples on the Couch

Following the critically acclaimed *Couples on the Couch: Psychoanalytic couple psychotherapy and the Tavistock model*, this volume offers further compelling ideas about couple psychotherapy from a psychoanalytic perspective.

The book well represents the foundational basis of the Tavistock Model and draws deeply from the work of Freud, Klein, Bion, Meltzer, and the contemporary Kleinians, while expanding the theoretical model by featuring ideas about couple relationships written from a variety of psychoanalytic frameworks. These additional frameworks include Winnicottian Theory, Fairbairn's Object Relations Theory, Link Theory, Self Psychology, Attachment Theory, Mentalization Theory, and Contemporary Relational Theory. This rich array of theoretical models, presented with exemplifying clinical material, results in a diverse assembly of papers that offer the reader an in-depth and complex view of a psychoanalytic approach to understanding and working with the dynamics of couple relationships.

With clear clinical guidance, this book will be invaluable for all psychoanalysts and psychotherapists working with couples.

**Shelley Nathans** is on the faculties of the Psychoanalytic Couple Psychotherapy Group and The Psychoanalytic Institute of Northern California and is director/producer of the film *Robert Wallerstein: 65 Years at the Center of Psychoanalysis*. Her publications include, "Oedipus for Everyone: Revitalizing the Model for LBGTQ Couples and Single Parent Families" (*Psychoanalytic Dialogues*, 2021). She is co-editor (with Milton Schaefer) of *Couples on the Couch: Psychoanalytic Couple Psychotherapy and the Tavistock Model* (Routledge, 2017). She is in private practice in San Francisco and Oakland, California.

# Relational Perspectives Book Series

Adrienne Harris,
Steven Kuchuck & Eyal Rozmarin
Series Editors

Stephen Mitchell
Founding Editor

Lewis Aron
Editor Emeritus

The Relational Perspectives Book Series (RPBS) publishes books that grow out of or contribute to the relational tradition in contemporary psychoanalysis. The term *relational psychoanalysis* was first used by Greenberg and Mitchell[1] to bridge the traditions of inter-personal relations, as developed within interpersonal psychoanalysis and object relations, as developed within contemporary British theory. But, under the seminal work of the late Stephen A. Mitchell, the term *relational psychoanalysis* grew and began to accrue to itself many other influences and developments. Various tributaries—interpersonal psycho-analysis, object relations theory, Self Psychology, empirical infancy research, feminism, queer theory, sociocultural studies, and elements of contemporary Freudian and Kleinian thought—flow into this tradition, which understands relational configurations between self and others, both real and fantasied, as the primary subject of psychoanalytic investigation.

We refer to the relational tradition, rather than to a relational school, to highlight that we are identifying a trend, a tendency within contemporary psychoanalysis, not a more formally organised or coherent school or system of beliefs. Our use of the term *relational* signifies a dimension of theory and practice that has become salient across the wide spectrum of con-temporary psychoanalysis. Now under the editorial supervision of Adrienne Harris, Steven Kuchuck, and Eyal Rozmarin, the Relational Perspectives Book Series originated in 1990 under the editorial eye of the late Stephen A. Mitchell. Mitchell was the most prolific and influential of the originators of the relational tradition. Committed to dialogue among psy-choanalysts, he abhorred the authoritarianism that dictated adherence to a rigid set of beliefs or technical restrictions. He championed open discussion, comparative and integrative approaches, and promoted new voices across the generations. Mitchell was later joined by the late Lewis Aron, also a visionary and influential writer, teacher, and leading thinker in rela-tional psychoanalysis.

Included in the Relational Perspectives Book Series are authors and works that come from within the relational tradition, those that extend and develop that tradition, and works that critique relational approaches or compare and contrast them with alternative points of view. The series includes our most distinguished senior psychoanalysts, along with younger contributors who bring fresh vision. Our aim is to enable a deepening of relational thinking while reaching across disciplinary and social boundaries in order to foster an inclusive and international literature.

A full list of titles in this series is available at https://www.routledge.com/Relational-Perspectives-Book-Series/book-series/LEARPBS.

## Note

1 Greenberg, J. & Mitchell, S. (1983). *Object relations in psychoanalytic theory*. Cambridge, MA: Harvard University Press.

# More About Couples on the Couch

Approaching Psychoanalytic Couple
Psychotherapy from an Expanded
Perspective

Edited by Shelley Nathans

Routledge
Taylor & Francis Group
LONDON AND NEW YORK

Cover image: Janoon028; iStock Photo, Getty Images

First published 2023
by Routledge
4 Park Square, Milton Park, Abingdon, Oxon OX14 4RN

and by Routledge
605 Third Avenue, New York, NY 10158

*Routledge is an imprint of the Taylor & Francis Group, an Informa business*

*British Library Cataloguing-in-Publication Data*
A catalogue record for this book is available from the British Library

ISBN: 978-1-032-20744-5 (hbk)
ISBN: 978-1-032-20745-2 (pbk)
ISBN: 978-1-003-26502-3 (ebk)

DOI: 10.4324/9781003265023

Typeset in Times New Roman
by SPi Technologies India Pvt Ltd (Straive)

For my loving family, Sam Gerson, Mara Nathans Gerson, and Nina Nathans Gerson

# Contents

# Preface

*Shelley Nathans*

The papers in this book and their accompanying discussions offer the reader an opportunity to explore the rich theoretical and clinical landscape of psychoanalytic couple psychotherapy. *More About Couples on the Couch: Psychoanalytic Couple Psychotherapy from an Expanded Perspective*, is the second volume in this series. The first book, entitled *Couples on the Couch: Psychoanalytic Couple Psychotherapy and the Tavistock Model*, primarily represents authors who worked from the model developed in London at the Tavistock Centre for Couple Relationships, now called Tavistock Relationships. The introduction in the first book will be useful to readers who seek an introduction to the history, theory, and core concepts that are cornerstones of the Tavistock model (Nathans and Schaefer, 2017).

This current volume, *More About Couples on the Couch*, also relies heavily on the Tavistock model and highlights its many important and foundational contributions. Readers will readily grasp how the Tavistock model has been influenced by Freud, Klein, Bion, and the contemporary British Object Relations theorists such as Britton, Steiner, and Joseph. The current volume presents a broader theoretical range, one that reflects an expanded psychoanalytic perspective of couple psychotherapy beyond the Tavistock model. Included are the contributions of Fairbairn, Winnicott, Bollas, Ogden, Field Theory, Mentalization Theory, Relational Theory, Self Psychology, and Link Theory.

The first volume of *Couples on the Couch* contains papers and discussions that were presented from 2008 to 2014 at the Annual Psychoanalytic Couple Psychotherapy Lecture, held in the San Francisco Bay Area. This popular and widely respected annual lecture series, co-hosted by the Psychoanalytic Couple Psychotherapy Group

(PCPG) and the Northern California Society for Psychoanalytic Psychotherapy, brings renowned international scholars to the San Francisco Bay Area to present original papers. Each paper is followed by a formal discussion given by a local Bay Area clinician and a subsequent clinical case presentation. The second volume in this series, *More About Couples on the Couch*, includes papers and discussions that were presented at the Annual Psychoanalytic Couple Psychotherapy Lecture, as well as papers intended to give the reader a broader exposure to the breadth of psychoanalytic couple psychotherapy, both in terms of topical content and theoretical range. Descriptive clinical material is included in the papers and this will help elucidate the unique theoretical and technical emphasis of each of these various models.

Volume 2 begins and ends with an important corrective to the long-neglected contributions of Winnicottian Theory to the psychoanalytic couple psychotherapy canon. The first four chapters use Winnicott to re-examine important themes in couple relationships. David Hewison's chapter, "Creativity and imagination in couple psychoanalysis: The influence of Winnicott and Bollas in clinical practice" (Chapter 1), presents the contributions of both Winnicott and Bollas and seeks to re-envision the previously dominant Kleinian and post-Kleinian model of creativity in couple relationships. In order to foster creative clinical work with couples, he discusses the technical implications of his thinking in the domains of gesture, repetition, compliance, mood, emotional atmosphere, and the use of objects. Shawnee Cuzzillo (Chapter 2), a practising artist and couple psychotherapist, discusses Hewison's paper by elaborating his departure from Klein's views of creativity. She discusses visual art as an analogy to highlight how the complexities of different points of view may be creatively brought together in both a painting and a clinical treatment.

In Chapter 3, "Love as creative illusion," Julie Friend approaches the topic of love – a surprisingly neglected topic in both psychoanalysis and in the psychoanalytic couple psychotherapy literature – as an inherently creative psychic state, one not necessarily realistically based or located in mature depressive position capacities but arising during emotionally intense currents that bear developmental potential. She uses Winnicott and other theorists to argue for a conception of love as a creative illusion – a state embodying emotional elements that includes less rational, creative, and aesthetic qualities that warrant our clinical attention. In her discussion of Friend's paper, Rachael Peltz (Chapter 4), elaborates Friend's argument for considering love in a separate register, and she locates it within a contemporary trend that focuses on what she calls "the ground" – the aspects of clinical work that attend to non-representational states and embodied dimensions that lead to a different form of communication and active engagement.

In my own chapter, "Infidelity as manic defence" (Chapter 5), I rely on a contemporary Kleinian model to explore some important themes that may underlie infidelity in the couple relationship. The paper focuses on the inability that one or both partners in a couple may have with mourning past or impending loss, and the consequent infidelity that may arise from a manic attempt to replace depression or psychic pain with excitement. In her discussion of my paper, Mary Morgan (Chapter 6) extends the focus to the couple's loss to the Oedipal situation itself – to the painful loss of their idealised primary objects and to the feeling of betrayal that comes with the awareness that there had been another idealised relationship that existed alongside the primary object's adult partner.

Amita Seghal's paper, "Viewing the absence of sex from the 'core complex' lens" (Chapter 7), attempts to understand the absence of sex in intimate relationships from a pre-Oedipal perspective. She provides a summary of different models that have been used to understand this symptom that is so frequently presented in couple psychotherapy. She uses Glasser's concept of the "core complex" to describe how unconscious claustro-agorophobic anxieties can be evoked about sexual contact and may underlie sexual difficulties for some couples. James Poulton offers a discussion of Seghal's paper (Chapter 8) in which he views the absence of sex in couple relationships from a broader perspective, as arising from a dialectical interaction on multiple dimensions stemming from different developmental phases, including Oedipal anxieties and the separate and shared unconscious representations of the internal couple in the partners.

In Chapter 8, "Lesbian and gay couple relationships: When internalised homophobia gets in the way of couple creativity," Leezah Hertzmann examines the relationship between desire and the potentially destructive impact of internalised homophobia that can produce a sense of paralysis in both the therapist and the couple. Hertzmann conceptualises the internalisation of homophobia in terms of superego development and argues that clinicians' unconscious biases may underlie countertransference reactions that can lead them to avoid making deep interpretations or talking about sex at all with lesbian and gay couples. Gary Grossman provides a cogent discussion that updates Hertzmann's study (originally published in 2011) in light of the political changes that have occurred in Western societies in the last decade as well as the theoretical developments in Hertzmann's own work – work that examines how disruptions in parental mirroring and Oedipal conflicts may have a particularly pernicious impact on those who later identify as gay or lesbian.

Molly Ludlam's paper, "Do Ronald Fairbairn's ideas still speak usefully to 21st-century couple therapists?" (Chapter 11), offers a clear introduction to Fairbairn's contributions to psychoanalytic theory, to the Tavistock model, and to couple psychotherapy. She makes a compelling case that his ideas are relevant for the contemporary psychoanalytic couple practitioner. In Chapter 12, Leora Benioff elaborates Fairbairn's object relations view with particular emphasis on the one-dimensional, rigid, and stereotypical nature of the unconscious representations that the partners in a relationship may cling to. Benioff usefully discusses some of the technical implications of approaching couple interactions with this model in mind.

Link Theory has greatly influenced the practice of psychoanalysis with individuals, couples, and families in Latin America, but because most of this literature has not been translated from Spanish, it has not been widely available to English-speaking clinicians. Monica Vorchheimer's paper, "Approaching couples through the lens of Link Theory" (Chapter 13), provides a rare and comprehensive introduction to this theory as it is applied to couple relationships. Link Theory expands the psychoanalytic frame beyond the historical dimension of the psyche, the body ego, the drives, and object relations by offering a perspective that subjects are also shaped by their links with others and their social environment – a model that is particularly apt as psychoanalysis attempts to integrate the influence of social, cultural, and political factors into our understanding of individuals and their relationships to others. In Chapter 14, Julie Friend offers an expanded discussion of both Link Theory and Vorchheimer's specific approach to working with couples – an approach that emphasises the alterity of the other and its impact such that, together, the couple is understood to form a new identity and a new unit of social structure. Friend situates this approach in relation to our familiar ways of understanding problematic couple dynamics and shows how Vorchheimer extends our view of the intolerance of difference beyond a theory of narcissistic relating.

Chapter 15 continues the expanded psychoanalytic perspective of this book with Carla Leone's study, "The application of contemporary Self Psychology to couple psychotherapy." This paper summarises contemporary Self Psychology's main contributions to understanding and treating couple relationships. Following Kohut, Leone highlights the importance of attunement to selfobject experience in couple therapy and advocates a point of view that understands dysfunctional behaviours as having a potential "forward edge." Rachel Cooke's discussion (Chapter 16) offers a brief history of Self Psychology and a summary of the differences between Leone's Self Psychological model and the Tavistock approach to working with couples. Cooke focuses on the theory of narcissistic relating – a central idea in the Tavistock model – and advocates that technical interventions beyond empathic attunement may be necessary when working with extremely narcissistic individuals in couple treatment.

The final two chapters of this book address endings. Taken together, they contribute an in-depth, psychoanalytic understanding of the difficulties inherent to working with high-conflict separating and divorcing couples. Chapter 17, "The co-parenting couple: Psychoanalytic technique with high conflict separating and divorcing couples," by Dana Iscoff, describes a model that enables the promotion of containment, reduces splitting, destructive aggression, and defensive projection. Further, her method strives to help the partners become more psychologically separate, enabling access to feelings of loss. Her technique relies on the development of a parenting plan that is used to facilitate the psychological development of the individual partners in order to help them transition from a separating or divorcing couple to a co-parenting couple. Avi Schmuli's discussion draws our attention to three domains: the necessary re-orientation of the separating or divorcing couple; the provision of hope in the assumption of development; and the projection of the children from the parent's projections.

I am confident that the readers of *More About Couples on the Couch: Approaching Psychoanalytic Couple Psychotherapy from an Expanded Perspective* will find a rich trove of clinically useful papers in this volume.

Like the first volume of *Couples on the Couch*, this book will provide both new and experienced clinicians with an in-depth, analytic approach to thinking about and working with couples and their relational difficulties. While still steadfastly rooted in the Tavistock model, the current book broadens the perspective and offers exposure to a variety of psychoanalytic models of couple psychotherapy. These papers, the discussions, and the clinical material that is offered in each of the chapters can enrich our theoretical understanding, enhance our clinical capacity, and help all of us who endeavour to work in this complex and challenging domain.

# Acknowledgements

I have been fortunate to have had the encouragement and support of family, friends, and colleagues while working on this project. To begin, I would like to express my gratitude to the authors of the papers and discussions in this book. I have learned a great deal from each of their distinct perspectives, analytic acumen, and scholarly contributions which collectively give this volume its extensive theoretical and clinical value.

I have benefited greatly from my participation in several professional communities, each of which has supported my development as a clinician, educator, and scholar. I am especially grateful to my fellow founders of the Psychoanalytic Couple Psychotherapy Group (PCPG). Leora Benioff, Rachel Cooke, Julie Friend, Milton Schaefer, and Sandra Seidlitz have been steadfast colleagues and collaborators – my thought partners. We have worked together for many years to create a vibrant home for psychoanalytic couple psychotherapy, scholarship, and training in the San Francisco Bay Area. This book would not have been possible without them or without my other PCPG colleagues with whom I share a passion for the study and practice of psychoanalytic couple psychotherapy.

It has been a privilege to be associated for many years with colleagues at Tavistock Relationships (formerly known as the Tavistock Centre for Couple Relations). I would particularly like to thank Mary Morgan, Stanley Ruszczynski, Chris Clulow, Francis Grier, Susana Abse, Andrew Balfour, David Hewison, and the late James Fisher for everything they have taught me. The training and theoretical model they have provided has served as a foundation for me in my development as a couple psychotherapist and for the content of this book.

I am grateful to the members of the Semi-Baked writing group (started by Judy and Bob Wallerstein) for their many years of colleagueship and for reading my work, including an early draft of my chapter, "Infidelity as manic defence" (Chapter 5 in this volume). Writing is not always an easy endeavour and I have appreciated having access to the minds of others who are also striving to commit their ideas to paper. I thank the Semi-Bakers: Ric Almond, the late Barbara Almond, Joseph Caston, Terry Becker, Daphne DeMarneffe, Dianne Elise, Sam Gerson, Peter Goldberg, Barbara Hauser, Laura Klein Markman, Henry Markman, Deborah Melman, the late Harvey Peskin, Tsipora Peskin, Rachel Peltz, Carolyn Wilson, and Mitchell Wilson.

Milton Schaefer was my co-editor for the first volume of *Couples on the Couch* (2017). I am indebted to him for his wisdom and dedicated work on the first book, without which this current project would not be possible. I am grateful to Lisa Buchberg and Ralph Kaywin for many thoughtful discussions about psychoanalysis, for reading my papers, and for generously providing careful editing. Julie Friend has provided insightful and helpful commentary on many of my scholarly papers. Beth Roosa has been a constant source of friendship and wisdom. I have been blessed to have many other friends and colleagues who have provided different types of support and encouragement over the years. I would like to express my gratitude to the following colleagues for their support: the late Lew Aron, Noa Ashman, Galit Atlas, Vivian Eskin, Jenn Guittard, Adrienne Harris, Hazel Ipp, Ortal Kirson-Trilling, Joyce Lindenbaum, Joyce Lowenstein, Damian McCann, James Poulton, and Monica Vorchheimer.

Thank you to my colleagues at the journals, fort da and Couple and Family Psychoanalysis, where many of the papers included in this book were previously published. In particular, I want to acknowledge Chris Clulow, Molly Ludlam, Alan Kubler, Patricia Marra, and Peter Silen. Thank you to the many fine people at Routledge who helped bring this book to publication: my editor Kate Hawes, her editorial assistant Georgina Clutterbuck, Thivya Vasudevan and the others who provided editorial and production support.

My daughters, Mara Nathans Gerson and Nina Nathans Gerson, have been boundless sources of encouragement. I am in awe of the dedication and passion that they each bring to life's endeavours and I am grateful for their loving spirits. My devoted husband, Sam Gerson, is my emotional bedrock, my source of intellectual inspiration, and my partner in all things. I thank him for his humour, support, and the loving life we have created together.

I want to sincerely thank my patients from whom I have learned so much. They each bring their vulnerabilities and strengths to my office, dedicating and rededicating themselves to this most unusual, yet undeniably special undertaking called couple psychotherapy.

# Credits list

The authors also gratefully acknowledge the permission provided to reproduce the following material:

"Re-visioning creativity in couple psychoanalysis: the importance of Winnicott and Bollas in clinical practice" by David Hewison was originally published in 2019 in *Couple and Family Psychoanalysis, 9(2)*: 167–180. Reproduced by kind permission of Phoenix Publishing House.

"Love as creative illusion and its place in psychoanalytic couple psychotherapy" by Julie Friend was originally published in 2013 in *Couple and Family Psychoanalysis 2(1)*: 3–14. Reproduced by kind permission of Phoenix Publishing House.

"Infidelity as manic defence" by Shelley Nathans was originally published in 2012 in *Couple and Family Psychoanalysis 2(2)*: 165–180. Reproduced by kind permission of Phoenix Publishing House.

"Viewing the absence of sex in couple relationships from the 'core complex' lens" by Amita Sehgal was originally published in 2012 in *Couple and Family Psychoanalysis 2(2)*: 149–164. Reproduced by kind permission of Phoenix Publishing House.

"Lesbian and gay couple relationships: When internalised homophobia gets in the way of couple creativity," Leezah Hertzmann, *Psychoanalytic Psychotherapy* 24(4): 346–360, © The Association for Psychoanalytic Psychotherapy in the NHS, reprinted by permission of Taylor & Francis Ltd, http://www.tandfonline.com on behalf of The Association for Psychoanalytic Psychotherapy in the NHS.

"Lost – and found – in translation" by Molly Ludlam was originally published in 2016 in *Fort Da: The Journal of the Northern California Society for Psychoanalytic Psychology XXII(2)*: 12–26. Reproduced by kind permission of Peter Silen.

"Response to Molly Ludlam's 'Lost – and found – in translation'" by Leora Benioff was originally published in 2016 in *Fort Da: The Journal of the Northern California Society for Psychoanalytic Psychology XXII(2)*: 27–36. Reproduced by kind permission of Peter Silen.

"Approaching couples through the lens of Link Theory" by Monica Vorchheimer was originally published in 2017 in *Fort Da: The Journal of the Northern California Society for Psychoanalytic Psychology XXIII(2)*: 17–30. Reproduced by kind permission of Peter Silen.

"Discussion of Monica Vorchheimer's 'Approaching couples through the lens of Link Theory'" by Julie Friend was originally published in 2017 in *Fort Da: The Journal of the Northern California Society for Psychoanalytic Psychology XXIII(2)*: 31–40. Reproduced by kind permission of Peter Silen.

"The application of contemporary Self Psychology to couple therapy" by Carla Leone was originally published in 2021 in *Couple and Family Psychoanalysis, 11(2)*: 170–186. Reproduced by kind permission of Phoenix Publishing House.

"Co-parent therapy and the parenting plan as transitional phenomena: Working psychoanalytically with high-conflict separating and divorcing couples" by Dana Iscoff was originally published in 2021 in *Couple and Family Psychoanalysis, 11(1)*: 14–26. Reproduced by kind permission of Phoenix Publishing House.

# Contributors

**Leora Benioff** has a practice in psychoanalysis and couple psychotherapy in Berkeley, California. She is a training analyst and faculty member at the San Francisco Center for Psychoanalysis and is a founding member and faculty at the Psychoanalytic Couple Psychotherapy Group in Berkeley. She is the North American co-chair of the IPA Committee on Couple and Family Psychoanalysis. She has presented on various topics relating to psychoanalytic couple therapy at multiple IPA conferences in the United States, Europe, and Asia. She has published in Couple and Family Psychoanalysis and Fort-Da, and contributed a chapter to the book, *Couples on the Couch: Psychanalytic Couple Psychotherapy and the Tavistock Model* (Nathans & Schaefer, 2017).

**Rachel Cooke** is a clinical psychologist in private practice in Oakland and San Francisco (on Zoom since COVID-19). She sees couples and individuals and provides consultation to therapists on working psychoanalytically with couples. She is a founding and faculty member of the San Francisco Bay Area's Psychoanalytic Couple Psychotherapy Group (PCPG) and has taught courses in psychoanalytic couple therapy at various other training programmes in the San Francisco Bay Area. She presented two papers at the COFAP conference of the IPA in San Francisco in February 2019. Her discussion of Stanley Ruszczynski's paper, "Couples on the Couch," was published in the book of the same name (Nathans & Schaefer, 2017).

**Shawnee Cuzzillo** is a psychoanalytically oriented psychologist, sees individuals and couples in Berkeley, CA, and supervises for community agencies in the San Francisco Bay Area. Dr. Cuzzillo is a graduate of the University of California at Berkeley, the Massachusetts Institute of Technology, the Wright Institute, and the Psychoanalytic Couple Psychotherapy Training Program. Her publications include papers on the intersection of evolutionary biology and psychopathology, and creativity in psychotherapeutic work. She teaches and supervises at graduate level and maintains an active art practice in her time outside the consulting room.

**Julie Friend** is a Board member of the Psychoanalytic Couple Psychotherapy Group and has served as Director of PCPG's Intensive Study Program since 2010. She serves on the Editorial Board of *Couple and Family Psychoanalysis*, is a member of Section VIII of Division 39 and has taught, supervised, and offered presentations on couple psychotherapy at many institutions. Her publications include, "Love as creative illusion and its place in psychoanalytic couple psychotherapy" (*Couple and Family Psychoanalysis*, 2013), and "Creative Illusion in couples: Thoughts about the value of transitional experience for couple relationships" (*Couple and Family Psychoanalysis*, 2021). She has a particular interest in Middle School thinking. Her private practice is in Berkeley, California, where she sees individuals, couples, and offers consultation.

**Gary Grossman** is a clinical psychologist and psychoanalyst in private practice in San Francisco, where he works with individuals and couples. He is a Training and Supervising Analyst at the San Francisco Center for Psychoanalysis, where he also chairs the Psychoanalytic Education Division, and is a Clinical Professor of Psychiatry and Behavioral Sciences at the University of California, San Francisco. He chaired the Committee on Gay & Lesbian Issues (now known as the Committee on Gender & Sexuality) of the American Psychoanalytic Association from 2000 to 2005, and served on that committee through 2016. He has been actively involved in teaching contemporary psychoanalytic perspectives for understanding the lived experiences of gay men and lesbians for over 30 years.

**Leezah Hertzmann** is a senior couple and individual psychoanalytic psychotherapist at the Tavistock and Portman NHS Foundation Trust (London, UK) and in private practice. She has a career-long interest in psychoanalytic theory and technique with LGBTQI individuals and couples and is a member of the British Psychoanalytic Council special advisory group on sexual and gender diversity. Recently, Leezah was the recipient of two British Psychoanalytic Council awards: firstly, for innovation in relation to her work with couples in dysregulated/violent relationships (2015), and the second (2019), the Bernard Ratigan Diversity Award, for developing and influencing psychoanalytic institutions towards a more inclusive sexual and gender-diversity culture. Leezah teaches and publishes widely and her most recent publication, authored with Juliet Newbigin, *Sexuality and Gender Now: Moving Beyond Heteronormativity*, is published by Routledge in the Tavistock Clinic Series.

**David Hewison** holds a doctorate in couple psychoanalytic psycho-therapy and is currently a consultant couple psychotherapist at Tavistock Relationships in London where he is head of research and ethics and runs psychoanalytic training. He is also a Jungian Training Analyst of the Society of Analytical Psychology and a member of the International Association for Analytical Psychology. He has a long-standing interest in links between psychoanalysis and Jungian analysis, with a focus on creativity and the imagination. He publishes widely and teaches internationally.

**Dana Iscoff** is a licensed Marriage and Family Therapist in private practice in San Francisco. She works extensively with separat-ing and divorcing families where she provides co-parent therapy, family therapy, reunification therapy, and individual therapy and coaching. She has been appointed as a Special Master/Parent Coordinator and Recommending Mediator, has conducted Child Custody Evaluations and Brief Focused Assessments, has worked as an expert witness, and has provided consultation to attorneys and community agencies on child custody matters. She has taught at the Family Law Section of the San Francisco Bar Association, the San Francisco Psychoanalytic Center and the Psychoanalytic Couple Psychotherapy Group. Her paper, "The parenting plan as transitional phenomena: working with high-conflict separating and divorcing couples," appeared in *Couple and Family Psychoanalysis*, 2021.

**Carla Leone** is the director of a group private practice just outside of Chicago, and on the faculty of the Chicago Psychoanalytic Institute and the Institute for Clinical Social Work in Chicago. She directs a certificate programme in Integrative Psychoanalytic Couple Therapy that is co-sponsored by both institutions. She is also Secretary of the International Association for Psychoanalytic Self Psychology (IAPSP), co-chairs its Membership Committee and its Online Education Committee, and co-founded IAPSP's Couples Therapy Interest Group and chaired it for many years. She is the author of several published papers on couple and family therapy and one on the "unseen spouse" of patients in individual therapy, and is cur-rently working on a book, tentatively titled *Rebuilding Connections, Repairing Ruptures: A Self Psychological Couple Therapy Casebook*.

**Molly Ludlam** is a couple and individual psychoanalytic psychotherapist. Now retired from clinical practice, she continues to enjoy
consulting, teaching, and writing. She is an author and editor of
several publications, including, *Couple Attachments*, co-edited
with V. Nyberg (Karnac,2007); *Couple and Family Psychoanalysis*
(founding editor 2011–2019); and most recently, "Can the 'internal couple' be our faithful life-long partner?", *Couple and Family
Psychoanalysis*,10(2): *1–29*. She is an external examiner at Tavistock
Relationships and the Tavistock Centre.

**Mary Morgan** is a psychoanalyst and couple psychoanalytic psychotherapist. She is a Fellow of the British Psychoanalytic Society,
Senior Fellow of Tavistock Relationships, Honorary Member of the
Polish Psychoanalytic Society and Consultant to the IPA Committee
of Couple and Family Psychoanalysis. She has contributed many
key articles and chapters in the field of couple psychoanalysis and
her recent book is *A Couple State of Mind: Couple Psychoanalysis
and the Tavistock Relationships Model*. She teaches and supervises
internationally and has a private psychoanalytic practice.

**Shelley Nathans** is on the faculties of The California Pacific Medical
Center, the Psychoanalytic Couple Psychotherapy Group, the
Psychoanalytic Institute of Northern California. She is the director
and producer of the film, *Robert Wallerstein: 65 Years at the Center
of Psychoanalysis*. She is on the international advisory board of the
journal, *Couple and Family Psychoanalysis* and is Chair of the Board
for the Psychoanalytic Couple Psychotherapy Group. Her most recent
publications include, "Oedipus for Everyone: Revitalizing the Model
for LBGTQ Couples and Single Parent Families"' (*Psychoanalytic
Dialogues*, 2021); "45 Years" (fort *da*, 2018); and "Whose Disgust is
it Anyway?: Projection and Projective Identification in the Couple
Relationship" (*Psychoanalytic Dialogues*, 2016). She is co-editor
(with Milton Schaefer) *of Couples on the Couch: Psychoanalytic
Couple Psychotherapy and the Tavistock Model* (Routledge, 2017).
She is in private practice in both San Francisco and Oakland,
California.

**Rachael Peltz** is Training and Supervising Analyst, Faculty member,
and Co-director of the Community Psychoanalysis Track at the
Psychoanalytic Institute of Northern California; and Supervising
Analyst at The Massachusetts Institute of Psychoanalysis. She is an
associate editor of *Psychoanalytic Dialogues*, and has published clinical papers on psychoanalytic listening, vitality, depth, the dialectic

of presence and absence, impasses in analytic couple work, and papers on the intersection between psyche and society including the manic society and a paper on refugee children suffering from resignation syndrome. She has a private practice in Berkeley, California and works with adults, adolescents, couples, and families.

**James Poulton** is a psychologist in private practice in Salt Lake City, Utah, an Adjunct Assistant Professor in Psychology at the University of Utah, and a member of the national faculty of the International Psychotherapy Institute (IPI). He currently is a member of IPI's Board of Directors, and serves on its Steering Committee. He has written extensively on psychological treatment and theory, with particular emphasis on a psychoanalytic approach to the treatment of couples. He is the author of *Object Relations and Relationality in Couple Therapy: Exploring the Middle Ground* (2012) and co-author of *Suffering and Sacrifice in the Clinical Encounter* (2020) and *Internalization: The Origin and Construction of Internal Reality* (2001). He has also co-authored two books on the history of art in the American West: *LeConte Stewart: Masterworks* (2012), and *Painters of Grand Teton National Park* (2015).

**Amita Sehgal** is a psychoanalytic couple psychotherapist accredited by the British Psychoanalytic Council (through the Tavistock Institute of Medical Psychology). She is a Visiting Lecturer at Tavistock Relationships and maintains a private practice in Central London where she sees individuals and couples. Her publications in the field of couple psychotherapy includes her edited book, *Sadism: Psychoanalytic Developmental Perspectives* (Karnac-Routledge, 2018). She has a special interest in the neurobiology of contemporary attachment perspectives in couple psychotherapy. Her ongoing interest in the psychological process of separation and divorce informs her commitment to resolving family disputes out of court, in a non-confrontational and constructive manner. She also consults with family lawyers, providing them with education, training, and bespoke services to maintain and optimise their performance and well-being.

**Avi Shmueli** is a psychoanalyst and couple psychoanalytic psychotherapist, having initially trained as a clinical psychologist and completed a research doctorate at UCL. He has worked in the UK's National Health Service, the Anna Freud Centre, and was a staff member at Tavistock Relationships for many years. He now works in private practice and supervises the work of the TR's Divorce and Separation Consultation Service. Committed to psychoanalysis as a theory for understanding the mind and as a mode of clinical practice, he has pursued its different applications, including empirical research and its application to the fields of both family and criminal law.

**Monica Vorchheimer** is a Training and Supervising Psychoanalyst at the Buenos Aires Psychoanalytical Association (APdeBA) and Member of the IPA and FEPAL. She has a private practice in Psychotherapy and Psychoanalysis with adolescents, adults, families, and couples in Buenos Aires, Argentina. She teaches and lectures locally and abroad as a Guest Professor in several places (Brazil, US., Russia, Israel, China). She is Co-Chair for Latin America at the IPA Committee on Psychoanalysis with Couples and Families (COFAP). Among her publications, she is Co-Editor with David Scharff of Clinical Dialogues on Families and Couples (Karnac, 2017).

Chapter 1

# Re-visioning creativity in couple psychoanalysis

## The importance of Winnicott and Bollas in clinical practice

*David Hewison*

My aim in this article is to focus attention on what I think is a compar-atively neglected area in contemporary couple psychoanalytic psycho-therapy: the work of Donald Winnicott and Christopher Bollas. Over the past decades, Kleinian and post-Kleinian thinking has been given more and more space in our writing and teaching with very fruitful results, but other voices have become muted – particularly those of the British Independent Tradition, which had been very much louder years ago. Couple therapists know that there is never only one way to think about things – different perspectives always have to be taken into account. This article is one of the ways in which the pluralism of the couple psychoanalytic psychotherapy field might be kept alive, and it makes a case for a re-visioning of creativity in our work. I think this re-visioning depends upon the capacity for clinical imagination – and I define this as, in effect, allowing thoughts and images and feelings to unfold in sessions, without shutting them down, concretising them, or fixing them in categories of what we already know. This necessi-tates more than one perspective. Obviously, this is not a new idea in psychoanalysis, but I am going to link it to a different conception of development and the role of the unconscious from that more usually found in the Tavistock Relationships model of couple psychotherapy.

I suggest that this model is incomplete because it leaves out the area of creativity that I am going to be discussing. The model, in effect, says that it is unconscious phantasy that links the couple, and that projection and projective identification are the dominant forces within the couple relationship. The idea is that we help couples understand the origins of these phantasies and withdraw these projections on each other. They can then become creative. As long ago as 1995, Warren Colman pointed out that there would be nothing keeping a couple

DOI: 10.4324/9781003265023-1

together in that case if therapy was successful. Kleinian and post-Kleinian ideas of creativity as relating to an internal couple have been vital in developing our contemporary psychoanalytic thinking about couple relationships (Morgan, 2018). However, Winnicott's criticisms of this, and Bollas' return to the creativity of dreamwork, suggest a wider view.

## The internal couple

Kleinian ideas of creativity and imagination, and their idea of an internal, heterosexual, parental couple as the foundation of mental health, suggest that creativity comes out of gratitude towards the internal parental couple and a wish to make reparation to them for the damage done to them in phantasy through envy and the work of the death drive (Klein, 1935; Money-Kyrle, 1971). Post-Kleinians such as Ron Britton usefully developed the idea of the couple in the mind when writing about how thinking can only arise when the capacity to be a third in relation to this internal couple is established, and when we can tolerate being excluded from their relationship, as well as, at times, excluding another from the relationship that we form (Britton, 1989). This idea of being the observer of a couple and being in a couple observed by another is important in couple psychotherapy – as it is in life. It forms a "triangular space" in which psychological life can mature. Couples have to relate to each other and to their relationship.

The concept of the internal, creative, parental couple undergoes a shift in our contemporary thinking to that of a "creative couple" in psychic space. Mary Morgan is responsible for extending this individual concept to a developmental achievement in couple relationships. The "creative couple" in the mind, in her idea, is simultaneously the property of each partner's internal world – stemming from the internalisation of the reality of a parental relationship that has survived Oedipal attack – and the property of the couple relationship itself, a shared unconscious phantasy that is deepened through relating (Morgan, 2005, 2018). The couple can use this internal connection to relate to each other and to take the strain of the external relationship when needed. What is additionally "creative" about this internal couple is that it is something that allows a coming-together of differences between the couple themselves in a way that can lead to something else. For example, where there is a blazing row between a couple, the shared phantasy of the creative couple between them allows for some sense of goodness in the relationship to be retained, even at the point when they are most furious with each other. Things are prevented from going too far or, if they do, are recovered from more quickly. Creativity, in this concept, includes the possibility of using another's mind (and allowing one's own mind to be used by the other) to create new thoughts and feelings. Morgan's concept is invaluable as a diagnostic aid when assessing a couple or thinking about how a couple therapy is going, and at times it is a state of mind that the couple therapist has to hold on behalf of a couple who are too disturbed or distressed to make use of it at any particular point.

So, in summary, creativity in this post-Kleinian view is a mix of reparative urges towards an object and the establishment of a state of mind in which innate benign coupling can be relied on. What might a Winnicottian view look like?

## Ideas of creativity: Winnicott

Winnicott was very clear about his position on creativity. Referring to the importance of Klein's development of the depressive position and the idea that creativity was a response by the baby to its destructive attacks on the mother, he said:

> In my opinion, however, Klein's important work does not reach to the subject of creativity itself and therefore it could easily have the effect of further obscuring the main issue.
>
> (Winnicott, 1971, p. 70)

The "main issue" that he is talking about is the relationship between the creative impulse and the environment. He goes on, having first dismissed the idea of the death instinct as merely a reassertion of original sin:

> We find either that individuals live creatively and feel that life is worth living or else that they cannot live creatively and are doubtful about the value of living. This variable in human beings is directly related to the quality and quantity of environmental provision at the beginning or in the early phases of each baby's living experience.

> Whereas every effort is made by analysts to describe the psychology of the individual and the dynamic processes of development and defence organisation, and to include impulse and drive in terms of the individual, here at this point where creativity either comes into being or does not come into being (or alternatively is lost) the theoretician must take the environment into account, and no statement that concerns the individual as an isolate can touch this central problem of the source of creativity.
>
> (Winnicott, 1971, p. 71)

Winnicott's use of the term "no statement" is absolute and is no respecter of psychoanalytic lineage – for him, neither Klein nor Freud get this right, and both are getting in the way.

For Winnicott, creativity was something primary, just as it was for Jung. It was not sublimation or restitution. It was not the consequence of the successful resolution of the Oedipal Situation, nor the establishment of the third position, though it necessarily influences all these. We can see that we are in a very different world when we view creativity from a Winnicottian perspective, as distinct from a post-Kleinian one. I think the differences are huge, not just in theory, but also in technique. There is also a difference in what we might think of as the "creative couple," in that Winnicott suggested this was the relationship between "being" and "doing," rather than mother and father, internal or otherwise.

If we think about Winnicott's idea of transitional space – something that is neither just an internal reality nor an external one – we can see that it belongs to the baby as well as to the mother. Even if something seems to be in the real world, its meaning is in the developing imagination of the infant. Winnicott talks of the necessity of not resolving this paradox too quickly: whether the baby makes it or finds it is something that must not be forced to a conclusion. While this links to ideas of reality testing, Winnicott is clear that it is not "reality" that needs to be built up in the child, but the capacity for play. Too quick an insistence on reality leads not to a true capacity to relate to oneself and the world, but to a "false self," in which imagination is sacrificed to an overly external-related position. Similarly, too little involvement of the world outside in the world of the infant leads to a schizoid or schizophrenic state, in which the real world is lost behind omnipotence, and the ability to be oneself is again lost. Winnicott writes of the demands of three kinds of worlds: the external world, the internal world, and the world of experience and illusion.

For Winnicott, being alive, in the fullest sense of the word, was creativity – he felt that the basic, good enough, developmental experience of the infant necessarily involved being creative. Creativity was the bedrock from which all else flowed. It was inherent in the baby but could only be made use of by virtue of the work of the mother in meeting the baby's omnipotent needs. It was as if the baby had created her, first facilitating the baby's illusion, and then gradually bringing-in disillusion, but at a pace that the baby could manage, thus mediating the baby's experience between inner and outer reality. As he put it:

> We have to say that the baby created the breast but could not have done so had the mother not come along with the breast at that moment: the communication to the baby is "Come at the world creatively, create the world: it is only what you create that has meaning for you." Next comes, "the world is in your control." From this initial *experience of omnipotence* that baby is able to begin to experience frustration and even to arrive one day at the other experience from omnipotence, that is to say having a sense of being a mere speck in the universe, in a universe that was there before the baby was conceived of and conceived by two parents who were enjoying each other.
>
> (Winnicott, 1987, p. 101)

Here, I think we can see Winnicott's response to the Kleinian idea that development comes from acknowledging the internal parents-in-intercourse and their supremely creative activity. It is clear that he sees it as part of development, and a necessary realisation, one that is to be hoped for, sought after as the opposite of omnipotence – "the other experience from" – and one that is at the end of a process of development that might even be arrived at "one day." This image of the parental couple having the baby in mind and then creating it themselves, in enjoyment of each other, is a highly complex one, and belongs to the depressive position (or as Winnicott preferred to call it, the "stage of concern") – something that he suggested was the *problem of life* for most people, not just the preserve of tiny babies (Winnicott, 1954).

This view suggests that creativity is not the product of an internal couple, that it does not stem from the acknowledgement of the facts of life as the Kleinians would say, but that it leads to the ability to acknowledge both the internal and the external couple – and indeed to become part of a couple oneself. Clinically, I think that this idea of the third area of experiencing means that when we hear about one member of a couple being destructive or dismissive, when they are projectively identifying an aspect of their internal world that they treat with disdain and attacking it in their partner, we also have to imaginatively grasp that this is an interaction in which a range of communications and demands are being made at the same time, by both partners, and that they are not only destructive or defensive. One partner's screaming at another that they are useless can also carry with it the wish that the other withstands this, or that they realise how useless the screaming partner feels and how unbearable it is, or even that they do, in fact, become less useless. The screaming can be a sign of hope, in addition to how we usually see it. Amidst the noise, there can be a creative move.

Winnicott suggests that this deep creative work is primary, helps us feel alive in the world, and that it goes on all the time in every aspect of life (unless we are ill, psychologically, and so unable to make use of it). Bollas takes this idea of the ongoing creativity of our interaction with the world and expands it radically and excitingly.

## Ideas of creativity: Bollas

Christopher Bollas is an American psychoanalyst who studied History at Berkeley in the 1960s and then English Literature in Buffalo. He trained clinically in the US and in London, where he lived for many years, and he is associated with the British Independent Tradition. His first book was *The Shadow of the Object* (Bollas, 1987). His latest is *Meaning and Melancholia*, which addresses the current state of social and cultural life in the age of Trump (Bollas, 2018).

Bollas' work is based on his deep reading of Freud – and particularly on those intuitions of Freud's that he was unable for one reason or another to develop. I shall set out some of Bollas' ideas that I find most helpful or evocative. This can only be schematic, but I hope that in the clinical examples I give later, the reader can get to see something of what they mean to me in practice. These ideas are the receptive unconscious, psychic genera, and psychic trauma, idiom and its relationship to the self, and the role of real objects. These concepts are all linked and his thinking about them is both multi-faceted and coherent.

Sarah Nettleton's (2017) introduction, *The Metapsychology of Christopher Bollas* is an excellent guide to his work.

## The receptive unconscious

Bollas draws upon Freud's highly sophisticated model of the unconscious found in *the Interpretation of Dreams* (Freud, 1900), in which processes other than repression are at work in the unconscious. In Freud's idea of dream work, we see a mix of unconscious perception, condensation, and representation. Freud says that the unconscious actively seeks out material during the experience of the day to give shape to itself during dreaming. In this process, the unconscious is highly creative and purposive. Bollas champions this view of the unconscious as actively at work perceiving, shaping, creating, and communicating in the most sophisticated way – indicating that this is a far cry from the idea of the unconscious as simply the depository of the repressed (Bollas, 2007). This perception requires us to accept that we do not know what is going on exactly in a couple's relationship. They are not only engaged in a process of projection or projective identification, which is the most common way of thinking about couple dynamics; they are making use of each other, at depth, in highly personal ways. But making use of each other to do what? This is where we need to think about the relationship between the innate creativity of the unconscious (what Bollas terms psychic genera) and its arch enemy: *psychic trauma*.

## Psychic genera and psychic trauma

Psychic genera are elements in the unconscious that gather together related ideas, images, and feelings, making links and creating new instances of each through building an ever-widening and sophisticated network of connections and associations in the mind, affecting consciousness (being capable of being known about) and generating a seeking-out of further similar experiences (Bollas, 1992). In this way, the unconscious gives rise to and shapes our conscious experience. Psychic genera reach out into the world and bring it back to us to be used in idiosyncratic ways depending on our personalities. We seek to make use of objects which are imbued with aspects of our unconscious through this process. These have entered the unconscious without being repressed because the unconscious is receptive; they have not been subject to symbolisation and so are "unthought knowns." The personality develops as more and more of these inner–outer experiences build up and link together. This is how Bollas sees the development of the mind and of thinking, and it is clear that it is more than just the tension between the reality and pleasure principles, life and death drives, triangular space, or solely the result of maternal containment. But what of psychic trauma, the opposite element in the psyche?

Typically, like Winnicott, Bollas focuses less on the wounding aspect of trauma, but more on the way in which the personality seeks to protect itself from the wound. Protection comes from shutting down the receptivity of the unconscious, making sure nothing similar gets in again. Networks of association are stunted, and nothingness is sought as the respite from pain; creativity is halted, and the outside world becomes a feared place. Trauma is a protective network that stifles; genera is a protective network that incubates, in order to intuit and allow something to form. This has clear implications for clinical technique: *it privileges waiting for emergence from within over interpretation from without*.

An example of this would be a couple I heard about in a supervision group in which the male partner was utterly unable to bear any links between his current relationship difficulties and his traumatic relationship with his mother. Attempts to show him how much he projected onto his partner were swiftly dismissed, and the therapist's comments about this dismissal simply became persecutions, rather than food for thought. The supervision group felt that the therapist should directly interpret his aggression and envy of another's mind, to get him to see what he was doing. I came to another conclusion, suggesting to the supervisee that she stop trying to get through to him, as she was getting caught up in the protective network of trauma that has to kill off thought. I felt that she should verbally note, in a factual way, when this refusal appeared – a bit like putting pins in a map – and then put a name to the area that the pins marked out, to the interaction when it happened again. We eventually settled on: "The area where my thoughts don't feel useful." When the situation repeated itself, the therapist would say, "We seem to be back in the area where my thoughts don't feel useful to you any more" and she gradually added riders like, "that must be hard" or, "that might feel quite a fragile thing." The name shortened to "The Area," and it became clear that it described an internal process, not just the particular interaction between the therapist and the couple. Slowly, this process began to be able to be talked about and the therapist could say things like, "The Area's at work again." Naming the phenomenon in this way, rather than insisting on interpreting it, allowed it to become a psychic genera, to move it slowly out of the grip of trauma, and enable it to accrete meaning again. It could then be talked about in couple terms: how it had been part of the fit between the partners, and how this enabled the female partner to hide her aggression in the problematic interaction between them.

### Idiom and its relationship to the self

Psychic genera – and by implication psychic trauma – are given unique shape by each person's unfolding and evolving personality, something Bollas calls "idiom" – our individual way of being that exists from the beginning like a kind of psychic fingerprint, an irreducible aspect of ourselves (Bollas, 1992). Idiom differs from Winnicott's "true self" in that it has robustness to it – it seeks out experiences where it can be manifest and met, though the degree to which it is free to do this depends on how well it was met in very early development. A mother who is free to discover who her baby is and can facilitate difference helps give form to the developing personality – one child might respond with pleasure and engagement to movements, another to sounds, and a third to shapes and textures. A well-attentive mother enables "aesthetic moments" in which a process of change occurs ("aesthetic" means "creative" in this context), a transformation from one state to another, in which what is important is the process of change, rather than the specific content. We relate to objects through their capacity to bring about transformation, to enable the linking of genera. Of course, this process is never complete and there are always elements of psychic trauma too, but the overall balance in the psyche depends on this meeting of unique personality and transformational experience. Bollas emphasises that, in this process, it is what the object does, rather than what the object is, that is important, and that our idiom also drives us towards our future. Idiom, rather than instinct, is what directs the psyche.

There is a similar quality to the self. Bollas describes this as the most complex of our psychic structures because it constantly shifts from one sense of self-experience to another. It represents different levels of awareness and different somatic, instinctual, and phantasy elements, involves relationships between our "day" conscious selves and our "night" dream working selves, and is most saturated by the unthought known. The self is distinct from the mind, and necessarily involves a split in the personality. Being a "self" is also a challenge to some people because it requires the ability to move between subjective and objective states, and because it is coloured by how we were seen and addressed by our parents when growing up (as Freud's concept of the superego suggests). Part of analytic work is to enable a more benign relationship between the self, in its many guises and qualities of experience, and the mind; to help those with whom we work to inhabit the self as it shifts and changes. The couple version of this benign relationship is where each partner has an active interest in the other's internal world – not as something to be threatened by and to control, but as something that brings new life into the relationship, something that can be used to develop the personality.

### The role of real objects

Because of the emphasis on process in Bollas' theory, the external world plays a much more important part in psychic development than it does in object relations theory. He suggests a key role for external objects and their effect on the personality, saying that the activity of the receptive unconscious means that external objects are constantly being sought out because of their capacity to transform idiom. These objects give rise to different trains of thought, act as symbols, represent a part of our history, and can be projected onto (Bollas, 1992). For example, the report in therapy of one partner's interest in a new colleague's sporting prowess may not only be envy or admiration, but can also indicate something about the missed pleasure of easily inhabiting the body, and when understood in this way, might lead to discussions about the couple's early sexual life, or issues about their ageing bodies.

### Technique

Bollas' view of the complexity of unconscious work has its counterpart in clinical technique. The idea of the innate creativity of the unconscious as the way in which the self manifests through idiom, seeking out and engaging with real external objects, as well as being shaped by internal ones, and by the impact of the as-yet unthought known, has clear implications for the clinical situation. Analytic technique is a coming-together of the creativity of both therapist and couple in a dialectic of difference. As such, it is important that we do not only tell the couple the unconscious meaning of their communications, but rather, that we work towards a situation in which the partners in the couple can become interested in, and curious about, their own unconscious minds, enjoy its complexity, and be open to being surprised by its actions. Our aim, following Winnicott and Bollas, is to encourage and support an experience in which the couple's unconscious is allowed more play in the couple's relationship. This requires more of the therapist's unconscious, more openness to association and imagination, and a not-knowing beforehand what the material refers to, let alone what it might mean. I consider there are five key areas that it is helpful for us to think about in terms of facilitating working in this way: gesture; repetition; compliance; mood and emotional atmosphere; and the use of objects.

### Gesture

The first requirement is that gesture is met properly. Winnicott likens gesture to the infant's use of aggression. He often talks of the "spontaneous gesture," and it is part of his description of the use of an object. The infant must be trying (aggressively) to use the object and destroy it in phantasy. The object must, simultaneously, survive this use and, by doing so, it comes to have real existence in the external world, and the infant becomes able to distinguish between fantasy and reality. In place of this aggression, considered as an essential element of the very young infants' finding themselves being alive, Winnicott sometimes spoke of "eagerness" (Winnicott et al., 1989, p. 240).

In Warren Colman's (1995) article, "Gesture and recognition as an alternative model to projective identification as a basis for couple relationships," he pointed out that couple therapy has to be about more than withdrawing projections. He proposed using Winnicott's connection between the baby's gesture and the mother's recognition, and response to it, as an alternative way of seeing what might otherwise be taken as problematic interactions between the couple, or between one or other partner and the therapist. Writing about a foursome therapy, he describes a split in the co-therapy pair, in which he responded differently to the partners from his co-therapist. Eric and Carole were a couple who had not had sufficient containment and holding in their early lives; they presented with very wearing violent emotional outbursts by Carole and defensive denial and withdrawal by Eric. This pattern continued in the consulting room, with no possibility of either partner containing the other's anxiety. Colman responded robustly to his perception of Carole's destructive attacks on the therapy and the relationship, whereas his co-therapist remained sympathetic to what she saw as an expression of a wish to be recognised and acknowledged. Colman suggested that he was responding not just to the original gesture, as his co-therapist was, but also to Carole's destructive defence against her own need when the original gesture had failed. Had the interpretation only ever been at the level of empathic maternal holding, Carole's aggression would have been denied and she would have been left hopeless that she could ever be truly found because the therapy would not be a robust enough setting for her. Instead, Colman's response, sometimes angry and forceful, gave her a sense of a boundary and then allowed her to make use of the softer, more enabling, intervention of the co-therapist. Gradually, the creative couple of the "being" and the "doing" of the co-therapy pair were more shared between them, matching the greater capacity of the couple to be in touch with themselves at the same time as being in touch with their partner.

### Repetition

We can see repetition not just as a compulsion, but as an ongoing attempt to find something new. If it is only interpreted as a historical remnant of a previous injury, the couple will be condemned to repeat it. For example, if a couple are persuaded that the distressing arguments they have when on holiday are best dealt with by carefully managing their time together, they will undoubtedly gain some relief in their relationship, but they will lose the opportunity to find whatever else it is that is being communicated in the fight. If the therapist is working well, s/he may do more than help them manage. She will make links to the partners' pasts, show them how they are repeating patterns from early childhood, and highlight how they are inducing and responding to incidents that do not belong to the present: mother was abandoning; father was intrusive. In this way, the couple can be helped to see that they not only respond to these perceived elements in their partner, but actively trigger them, and by doing so, they are performing an abandoning–intruding dance that is very wearing for all concerned. This technique can be helpful, projections are being identified and withdrawn, but it has limitations.

The problem is that the experience is in the present and that the interpretation assumes it does not belong there. If the couple recognise that their therapist is well-meaning, and if they are a couple who can feel concern and the value of reparation easily enough, they will work hard to adapt themselves to become the couple that the therapist seems to want them to be, knowing that this is probably going to be quite good for them. However, they can find themselves beginning to react to each other in familiar ways, and then clamp down on this reaction for the good of the relationship. An aspect of their emotional lives will become felt to be inauthentic and flat, and they will try to avoid noticing it as doing so will inevitably lead back to the original problem. I am suggesting, following both Winnicott and Bollas, that there is more to be understood in this repetition.

We could imagine the therapist and the couple coming to the brave realisation that the progress has been false in some way, that the interpretative work that led to the withdrawing of projections from each other has somehow missed the point. But what might this point be? A clue is in the idea that repetition is simply that: a repeating of what is already known in order to avoid the not-yet-known; it is not an elaboration or an expansion of associations. It could be said that the couple do not argue enough, that they have never really got through to each other, but that they have never faced what this failure means. Fortunately, they are beginning to know something about failure because of the realisation that the therapy has, so far, failed them. There is now a chance to explore what this is like, what meanings they give to it, how it makes them feel. The therapist needs to be interested and not defensive about this process. The fury at being failed by their parents and the pain of failing to keep struggling with their parents' failure and their part in it, then becomes the stuff of the therapy. The arguments stop being evacuations and become communications. The couple move from doing things to each other, to being with each other, and the repeated attempt to create the world so that it can be used, will no longer be missed. Psychic trauma will be replaced by psychic genera.

## Compliance

The kind of fitting-in that can happen when repetition does not find its true aim or when attempts to use the object through spontaneous gestures are rejected, can lead to compliance. Winnicott thought that this was amongst the worst things that could happen to a child, resulting in the development of a truly false caregiver, self. In Bollas' terms, the true idiom of the person is stunted, and the network of genera becomes limited.

Compliance is something that is particularly problematic in couple relationships because of the difficulty in managing the different pulls between closeness and distance, dependence and independence, that are required in committed partnerships. Couples where one partner insists on being right and is felt to be overwhelming, or the other puts up no resistance and so is felt to not be there, have this problem. In their different ways, both are attempting to force compliance – the one actively, the other passively.

Similarly, couples who try to live out ideals about relationships either passed down to them directly by parents, or indirectly by wanting to be who their parents were not, may have a problem with compliance – this time with an idea. For example, sometimes couples live through their children, trying to give them everything they feel they never had. This becomes problematic when it prevents the children having their own ideas about who they are and what they want, who find their parents suffocating, or who – rather than rebelling or protesting – come to have no mind of their own, sometimes to the extent of having a breakdown, which serves to legitimise the active role of the parents in the child's life. These couples need to be invited to have a different experience from the ideal and be helped to manage its demands.

Therapists also can unwittingly encourage compliance, especially when they continue down a line or style of interpretation that has its roots in a theoretical understanding of something like the Oedipus complex, without being open to nuance. The couple may be persuaded by the approximation of the interpretation, but also by their therapist's apparent inability to do anything different. If they protect the therapist and accept the interpretation, they give up themselves. This means that therapists always have to be open to questioning what they are doing with any couple, particularly when they find that they are doing the same kind of thing with all their cases.

## Mood and emotional atmosphere

Attending to these phenomena is not just as a way of trying to see what kind of object relationship is in play at any one time, in the usual way, but also what version of the self of either partner (or indeed what version of the couple self) is currently in play. This is difficult to track, and the therapist has to be able to tolerate the session unfolding without intervening, while attending to the ebb and flow of their own self-state, in order to allow something to coalesce. Sometimes this will mean stopping the partner interrupting, or just encouraging staying with an image or a feeling. In this kind of intervention, the aim is not to achieve an interpretation, but simply to allow something to be, for the unconscious to do its work. Being is more important than interpreting – "After being – doing and being done to. But first, being," as Winnicott put it (Winnicott, 1971). Here is an example:

A couple arrives for a session, each partner bringing an atmosphere: Erik is bouncy, anxious, constantly moving his gaze from me to Ivan and back again. Ivan is very still, and he seems to have a slight smile, as if contemptuous of Erik, me, and the therapy. I already know that they complain of a disapproving father–rebellious adolescent son dynamic between them, and at first sight this seems to be what is being brought today. Erik will make a claim for my support as a sensible grown-up, and Ivan will initially deny any accusation Erik makes and promise he will never do it again. I decide not to say anything, but to wait and see what happens. I notice a feeling of boredom and the sense of repetition. The conversation is all about how Ivan had promised not to stay out partying, but then did, leaving Erik waiting at home. Erik eventually deadlocked the door so that Ivan would not be able to get in, but Ivan had not noticed as he had not come home. Erik despairs, saying nothing he does makes any difference. Ivan seems livelier and his smile is broader, but there is something fixed about it. The atmosphere in the room has changed, and I am suddenly not bored. Curiously, I feel strongly present, and I know we are on the cusp of something. I say, as much to myself as to them, "What must it be like when a dead lock makes no difference?" My unvoiced thought is that ghosts pass through doors. Both partners are very still and quiet. Ivan lets out a slow sigh. We begin to talk for the first time about the death of his parents in the

Balkan conflict. The atmosphere in this and the following sessions changes to one of painful work as we explore both of their experiences of death, loss, hope, and guilt. They are no longer locked in with the dead, but able to open the door to the living relationship between them.

## Use of objects

The final area is the way in which we conceive of the couple's use of other people and other things. We need to be interested in descriptions of external events, people, and relationships, not simply as projections of internal states or object relationships, and particularly not as only descriptions of the transference relationship to the therapist, but also as possible instances of something new that can be used by either partner or the couple in the idiosyncratic service of development. Winnicott's idea of the blurred area between the child's imagination and the world beyond it carries with it the need not to demand too quickly that reality is put first. This matches Bollas' idea that the unconscious is selecting elements of reality to work within the service of idiom. We have to be open to recognising these descriptions as part of a pattern, instances of which are seen in other domains, such as accounts of history, the punchline of jokes in sessions, or the stumbling over certain words or phrases. It is the pattern perceptible in the narrative and its effects, rather than the narrative itself that is important.

Some years ago, I saw a couple in their early sixties who said that their relationship had been distant after their youngest child left home. Each of them had been busy and admitted that they had not spent much time together, nor had they cared about this over the years. She was part of a choir, and he did voluntary work as a financial administrator for a charity for the homeless. Nonetheless, they felt that something was missing between them. We had been able to see the ways in which her activities had, symbolically, given her a voice (she had grown up in an extremely controlling household) and that he had found a kind of help for his feeling of being homeless inside (having been sent to boarding school when he was seven).

One session, he reported feeling perturbed that something was not quite right in the financial ledgers in the charity, and he wondered whether some cheating was going on – though there seemed to be more, rather than less, money in the account than expected. This was a session in which the couple had been given a bill which included a session that they had missed because of severe weather. It was obvious that this could be taken up in terms of the couple's feeling cheated about having to pay for a session they had not had, but I decided to wait and see what else arose. She did not pay much attention to his story, but talked about what interested her: a friend in her choir was distressed because deteriorating eyesight meant that she was not quite able to read the sheet music and in particular could not tell what line the notes were on. They blurred together and it was all too much. It seemed to me there were anxieties about things not being right or failing.

They continued their parallel stories: he worried he might be wrongly blamed for the potential irregularities; she talked about how the choir would lose its value to her if her friend left. The stories came together as they each wondered whether or not they might have to leave these activities that absorbed their time. I pointed out that they might have to spend time together and they both laughed, with what I noticed was some relief. I wondered aloud whether the lines in which they had lived their lives (those of the financial ledger and in the sheet music) no longer served their purpose of guiding them and holding them to account as "right." I pointed out the too-muchness in their stories and suggested that something was going on for each of them simultaneously, and that I was not sure what it was. It just seemed as if they now had more to offer each other and that this might at long last be a relief. They accepted this, unsure about what was to them a new feeling, and aware that they needed help to make a new shared life together. The objects they had each used as a relief from the demand of relating to each other had developed them. As a result, they were each in a better place to relate to one other at the very point that their separate activities let them down in parallel. I am suggesting that this was no accident.

## Conclusion

To end my paper, I would like to reiterate my claim that there should be space in contemporary discussions about psychoanalytic work with couples for perspectives other than the post-Kleinian, which is becoming the default in psychoanalytic couple psychotherapy. Every theory is a form of perception. We need more than one way of making sense of what it means to relate to another, to help us find the humanity unfolding in the relationships between ourselves and our minds, with our others and our objects, and in the processes of being and doing inherent to creative coupling. The pictures of the psyche laid out by both Winnicott and Bollas are essential as a corrective, both theoretically and clinically, to our dominant model of couple psychoanalysis. In *The Mystery of Things* Bollas (1999) describes psychoanalytic work as an Oedipal Situation that involves three kinds of mental states: the maternal order of diffuse attention; the paternal function of focus and interpretation; and the infantile function of dream-like self-absorption. There can be no creativity without the openness of the third, beyond the creative couple, to the creative unknown of the unconscious in all its forms.

# References

Bollas, C. (1987). *The shadow of the object: Psychoanalysis of the unthought known*. London: Free Association Books.

Bollas, C. (1992). *Being a character. psychoanalysis and self experience*. London: Routledge.

Bollas, C. (1999). *The mystery of things*. London: Routledge.

Bollas, C. (2007). *The Freudian moment*. London: Karnac.

Bollas, C. (2018). *Meaning and melancholia: Life in the age of bewilderment*. Abingdon & New York: Routledge.

Britton, R. (1989). The missing link: Parental sexuality in the Oedipus complex. In: R. Britton, M. Feldman, & E. O'Shaughnessy (Eds.), *The Oedipus complex today: Clinical implications* (pp. 83–101). London: Karnac.

Colman, W. (1995). Gesture and recognition as an alternative model to projective identification as a basis for couple relationships. In: S. Ruszczynski & J. Fisher (Eds.), *Intrusiveness and intimacy in the couple* (pp. 59–73). London: Karnac.

Freud, S. (1900). *The interpretation of dreams*. S.E., 4: ix–627. London: Hogarth.

Klein, M. (1935). A contribution to the psychogenesis of manic-depressive states. *International Journal of Psycho-Analysis*, 16, 145–174.

Money-Kyrle, R. (1971). The aim of psychoanalysis. *International Journal of Psycho-Analysis*, 52, 103–106.

Morgan, M. (2005). On being able to be a couple: The importance of a "creative couple" in psychic life. In: F. Grier (Ed.), *Oedipus and the couple* (pp. 9–30). London: Karnac.

Morgan, M. (2018). *A couple state of mind: Psychoanalysis of couples and the Tavistock relationships model*. London: Routledge.

Nettleton, S. (2017). *The metapsychology of Christopher Bollas: An introduction*. Abingdon & New York: Routledge.

Winnicott, D. W. (1954). The depressive position in normal emotional development. In: *Through paediatrics to psycho-analysis: Collected papers* (pp. 262–277). London: Hogarth.

Winnicott, D. W. (1971). *Playing and reality*. London: Penguin.

Winnicott, D. W. (1987). *Babies and their mothers*. London: Free Association Books.

Winnicott, D. W., Winnicott, C., Shepard, R., & Davis, M. (1989). *D. W. Winnicott: Psycho-analytic explorations*. Cambridge, MA: Harvard University Press.

Chapter 2

# Discussion of "Re-visioning creativity in couple psychoanalysis"

## The importance of Winnicott and Bollas in clinical practice

*Shawnee Cuzzillo*

## Introduction

I am very pleased to have this opportunity to discuss David Hewison's paper. For Hewison, creativity is a primary drive, which challenges the wisdom of the historical reliance on Kleinian and Post-Kleinian theory as the bedrock of psychoanalytic couple work. He relies on Winnicott and Bollas to address these questions about creativity. His theoretical argument stands in contrast to the traditional Tavistock model, which typically views the origin of creativity as secondary, rather than primary. To oversimplify, for Freud, creativity is the product of the sublimation of sexual drives. For Klein, the source of creativity is in the reparative wish toward the internalised parental couple that, in phantasy, has suffered the child's primitive infantile and Oedipal attacks. Hewison contrasts these views of creativity with those of Bollas, Winnicott, and Jung, who see creativity as primary. Seeing the source of creativity as a primary impulse promises to inform Hewison's technique with couples. This offers a refreshing approach, based on viewing the psyche's efforts to grow creatively, despite what may seem, at first glance, like destructive or compulsive repetition. The essence of Hewison's contribution and the question he poses strikes at the heart of the matter: *If creativity is primary, if it is a primal, central drive and not secondary in human nature, how does this affect how we see couples; how we theorise about couples; and how we treat couples?*

A couple is a fantastically complicated system. I am always humbled by the awareness of how limited our vision is, and how few bits we can see, understand, or hold in mind at any given time about such a complex phenomenon. Sitting in a room with two human beings, who have a connection with one another that has been evolving over months or decades, while simultaneously engaging with both individuals and the couple, is a highly complex and dynamic process. We are

DOI: 10.4324/9781003265023-2

both witness and participant to psyches connected receptively and defensively. At the same time, projections are flying, projections are landing, and unconscious bargains are being made. Each member of the couple brings to the relationship a soup of phantasies, expectations, fears, wishes, and a desire for a transformational experience.

As Bollas states:

> Our minds are far too complex to be about any one thing, be it a repressed idea, an id derivative, the transference or anything. Indeed, at any moment in psychic time, if we could have a look at the unconscious symphony it would be a vast network of creative combinations.
>
> (Bollas, 2013, p. 27)

No wonder any one theoretical model that we apply to help us understand the complexity of couple relationships will be inherently limited. There are so many theories, or languages, we could use to describe what is going on between two people in a couple, and yet, we still would not capture the totality of what is happening. One of Hewison's major contributions in this study is to extend our capacity to understand these dynamics. In order to do this, he takes us out of our comfort zone by helping us think beyond and outside of the constructs of Kleinian and Post-Kleinian theories.

Hewison invites us on a quest to find a way to cultivate, within the therapist as well as within the couple, an atmosphere and set of technical approaches that are the most conducive to creative work. Work with couples, at its best, can both demand and elicit states of peak creativity in all three participants. At its worst moments, it can propel all three participants into dead and lifeless places where creativity of any kind seems impossible.

## Creativity

Hewison invites us on a quest to find a way to cultivate, within the therapist as well as within the couple, an atmosphere and set of technical approaches that are the most conducive to creative work. Work with couples, when at its best, can both demand and elicit states of peak creativity in all three participants. At its worst moments, it can propel all three into dead and lifeless places from which creativity seems to be impossible to develop.

Hewison cites Morgan's seminal work on the "couple state of mind," a key concept that has been used to understand how a creative couple functions and what is missing in those who are unable to create anything new. Morgan states that if the couple is shaky in their ability to use each other's minds creatively, it is incumbent upon the therapist to use her own mind to hold the differences in the couple and help them use these differences in a new way (Morgan, 2001). Hewison adds to this formulation by advocating an approach that facilitates the development of the primary creativity for all the individuals in the room, including the couple and therapist, which emphasises the importance of the therapist fostering an attitude that facilitates creativity. This orientation raises some fundamental questions. How do we work with ourselves internally to accomplish this? How do we foster the growth of therapists in our community to enhance creativity and imagination in their clinical work? How do we use theory and the structure of the psychoanalytic frame, while still maintaining an atmosphere that can receive a spontaneous gesture and promote creative responses to our patients?

## Polarities in creativity

I want to thank Hewison for his excellent summary of the literature on creativity in Winnicottian, Kleinian, and Post-Kleinian theory. While a full review of all the psychoanalytic literature on creativity is beyond the scope of this discussion, I do want to highlight two others that I think deserve mention because they also emphasise an area between polarities, an intermediate area, as central to creative potential.

Sylvano Arieti (1976) wrote about creativity from a Freudian perspective and coined the phrase "tertiary process" to describe the blend of primary and secondary processes required for creativity. Ernest Kris (1952) developed his idea of "regression in the service of the ego" as an attempt to bridge the polarities of regression with the aim of the mature ego. Although Arienti was grounded in Freudian theory and Kris in ego psychology, the centrality of the polarities in the psyche and the intermediate space necessary for creativity link them to both Winnicott and Hewison.

What types of polarities might we consider in relation to creativity? These psychic polarities might include: rational/irrational; inner/outer; intuition/logic; linear/nonlinear; conscious/unconscious; reality/phantasy; right brain/left brain; differentiation/merger; and primary/secondary process. As Hewison points out, Winnicott's (1971) concept of transitional space is also situated between internal and external reality and rests on the importance of not resolving these polarities prematurely in order for the imagination to develop.

This understanding of creative processes can be extended to aspects of emotional experience. Friend, applying Winnicottian theory to romantic love writes:

> ... love, at the very heart of couple relationships, is a state that is often far from realistic – it can be full of idealization, blurred boundaries, fantasy, and illusion. Is there a place in psychoanalytic psychotherapy with couples for listening on a separate register to the intense, non-reasonable emotional vicissitudes of love? Is it useful to consider balancing the emphasis on the value of mature, realistic relating with that of less rational, more embodied forms of relating in couples? How do we as couple psychotherapists hold a place for both, and help couples build their capacity to hold a tension between more mature, reasoned kinds of relating on the one hand, with the creative potential of less rational, more aesthetic qualities of relating to the other?
>
> (Friend, this volume p. 35)

Friend's idea of love, as a creative act, shares many qualities with Hewison's ideas about creativity. She makes an argument for finding love in the intermediate space that Winnicott describes, and she wonders whether too much insistence on "reality" in matters of love misses the point. Love and creative relating may, in fact, live most vitally in this intermediate area between reality and illusion. Friend's paper is a significant contribution in the direction of allowing the intermediate area of experience to be appropriately valued and honoured in our work with couples, and it creatively invites us to examine our own experience in this work.

## Art as analogy

An analogy in the realm of painting may be useful. In doing so, I am relying on the ideas of Winnicott, Bollas, Hewison and Morgan's (2001) concept of a "couple state of mind" to illustrate how both creating and viewing art rely on transitional space. These ideas bring to mind how I feel standing and looking at impressionist paintings, because they are such a lovely blend of the inner and outer worlds. As I am looking at a painting, I am thinking of the painter looking at a scene that was actual, outer reality, at a particular time and place. The perception of this scene, through the eyes and mind of the painter, was translated into choices of colour, placement, contrast, and the embodied movement of the paint brushes, to create a version of the scene that is uniquely influenced by the subjectivity of the painter. The painter is expressing her unique idiom through the medium of paint. Perhaps this is why one can recognise the distinctive idiom in a painter's work across paintings, or even across a large room in a museum; it's like spotting an old friend in the distance. At moments during a painting experience, there is a sense of being both at one with and separate from the scene.

Similarly, in a group of painters, in a figure painting class, the whole group is looking at the same figure in objective reality, but each one from a different angle or perspective. If you walk around in a class like that, it is delightful and surprising to see how strikingly different each painter's view of that objective scene will be. In my view, several polarities are being bridged in these experiences, including differentiation and merger, primary and secondary processes, inner and outer reality, and logic and intuition.

To fully appreciate how to understand the complexity of bridging these polarities within a couple therapy, the therapist must listen to a scene being painted differently by each member of the couple, and she must appreciate them equally. This is what Morgan means by a couple state of mind (Morgan, 2001). For the couple therapist to appreciate the scene being painted by each partner as a creative work, as a scene coloured both by both the perception of external reality and by the internal world, playful and inclusive communication about these two versions must be fostered. This is a far cry from what couples often appear to be asking us to do when they set us up to pick which version of the story is the correct version, when they attempt to make us be both judge and jury!

## Clinical imagination

Hewison defines clinical imagination as, "allowing thoughts and images to unfold in sessions, without shutting them down, concretizing them, or fixing them in categories of what we already know" (this volume, p. 1). His description of clinical imagination is resonant with Bion's idea that we approach each session "without memory or desire" and that we should strive to move between knowing and not knowing (K and –K) (Bion, 1963). Bion is encouraging us to hold both polarities, something between what we come to "know" about our patient, and the encounter with "ultimate reality" or "absolute truth," what he termed "O" (Bion, 1963). Delving deeply into Bion is beyond the scope of this discussion, but I want to highlight how this conception gives us a sense of the movement between the knowledge that a formulation provides, and the awe of the unknowable and mysterious aspects of both the universe and of the people we work with. This Bionian perspective is very consistent with the model Hewison presents in terms of encouraging the therapist to keep access to imagination alive in the treatment.

This use of imagination in psychoanalytic work is closely related to the art of cultivating the therapist's reverie and has been well elaborated by Ogden (2005). Ogden describes states of reverie as times when we let our minds have the freedom to wander into our own associations, with thoughts, feelings, and images, as they arise, to foster a more creative approach in our work with patients. Attending to our own reverie permits us to have more access to our unconscious as it bubbles up. Hopefully, our associations relate, to some extent, to what is happening unconsciously in our couples. In other words, we strive to use what arises in our own reverie as a possible window into what is happening in the unconscious, in the back-and-forth dynamics within the psyches of our couples. The practice of attending to our own reverie as a source of information can be challenging with an individual patient, but it can be much more difficult to achieve with a couple, especially one caught in the grip of a stormy conflict.

## Repetition

For Freud, the repetition compulsion was linked, at worst, to the death instinct, and at best, to an attempt to master painful past experiences. In "Beyond the Pleasure Principle," Freud (1922) described the fort da game. He described how a child delights at the repetition of a game in which he is clearly enjoying mastery over the disappearance and reappearance of objects. There is a special pleasure in the return of the object. Freud used this example to speculate and explain a variety of pleasures and repetitions in both child's play and in adult behaviour. Freud concluded that repetition may be a reflection of the death instinct, a concept which he defined as the tendency of all life to return to an inorganic state.

One of the most challenging, yet exciting aspects of Hewison's paper is his emphasis on the creative potential of the repetition compulsion. It is typical for psychoanalysts and psychotherapists to view repetitions as primarily destructive in nature, as anti-developmental activities (need references here). Hewison invites us to also see a creative edge and developmental possibility in these repetitions. To demonstrate this, he provides an analysis of a couple in a fight:

> One partner's screaming at another that they are useless can also carry with it the wish that the other withstand this, or even that they realise how useless the screaming partner feels and how unbearable it is, or even that they become less useless. The screaming can be a sign of hope, in addition to how we usually see it. It can be a creative move.
>
> (Hewison, this volume p. 6.)

While tolerating difficult repetitions is often taxing for both individual and couple therapists, the challenges when working with destructive repetitions in each of these settings differ. In individual treatment, it might be easier to withstand a patient's tantrum and then slowly work to help them find words to describe their emotional outburst. The therapist might even be able to help the patient develop the capacity to own the destructive, regressed parts that could only be communicated in this way, and ultimately, together they might find the beginnings of a true self within the tantrum. However, in the context of a couple treatment, we must also contend with the impact the tantrum is having on the other partner. The impact may be significant and so destructive that it can become imperative for the couple therapist to interrupt the screaming. The crucial technical dilemma in such a scenario is to find a way to intervene, to be responsive to both partners, that doesn't destroy what Hewison understands to have developmental potential, what he calls the "creative move."

Hewison is pointing to a *creative edge within the repetition compulsion*, which turns the usual way of thinking about the repetition compulsion on its head. In his way of thinking, something new is being created, and the true aim of the repetition that is creative and developmental. To take the screaming as a creative move would be challenging for the therapist, but also potentially highly effective in some instances. Essentially, Hewison may be saying, let's not put the pacifier in the mouth to stop the scream; let's really try to hear it in the most alive way, a way that includes creative development as part of the message in the scream. Hewison, following Winnicott and Bollas, is always looking for play, creativity, and development, even in the most apparently toxic interactions. But I wonder if there are repetitions that should be understood to be purely toxic? And if so, how do we tell the difference between creative repetitions and those that are not developmental in nature?

## Facilitating environment and technique

As Hewison points out, for Winnicott, creativity is a primary impulse, but it only comes into being *in the context of a facilitating environment*. Hewison's quotes from Winnicott's, *Playing and Reality* (Winnicott, 1971, p. 71): "...no statement that concerns the individual as an isolate can touch this central problem of the source of creativity." As the infant is not an isolate, neither is the adult. When individuals create couples and families, they are more or less able, depending on their own creative capacities, to co-create environments that foster creativity. Through a Winnicottian lens, Hewison helps us to see the importance of therapists providing creative, facilitating environments for all couples, but especially for those whose own creativity is impaired.

In thinking about technique, I would like to first highlight how creativity may be stifled in couple relationships. In some cases, according to Winnicott (1965), the individual partners may have had a failure in the early environmental conditions that led to a false self. Or, according to Bollas (1992), psychic trauma has shut down the receptivity of the unconscious. Hewison states, "protection comes from shutting down the receptivity of the unconscious, making sure nothing similar gets in again" (this volume, p. 8). For those couples in which a false self has developed, or when psychic trauma is significant, fostering a facilitating environment in the treatment will be crucial. But how do we do this and what is involved? What are the components of such a facilitating environment in our work with couples?

## Mood and atmosphere

As Hewison suggests, attending to the mood and atmosphere in the room with the couple is an important component of couple psychotherapy. Following Winnicott (1971), Hewison addresses this by emphasising the necessity of being sensitive to the mood of the couple and first responding by just "being." The quality of our "being" includes nonverbal communications that respond to the atmosphere between the couple and influence what might be possible between them. Depending on the couple, each facilitating environment will have a different flavour or rhythm. Like Winnicott's (1973) good-enough Mother who tunes herself to her child and adapts herself to what her child needs, we must tune ourselves to the unique needs of each couple.

## The use of objects and transitional space/compliance

Hewison's discussion of Winnicott's concept of the use of objects offers some refreshing ideas about how to listen to the patient's account of external events, and of the people in their lives. He suggests that we listen to these descriptions:

> ... as possible instances of something new that can be used by either partner or the couple in the idiosyncratic service of development. Winnicott's idea of the blurred area between imagination and the world beyond it carries with it the need not to demand too quickly that reality is put first.
>
> (Hewison, this volume, p. 16)

To illustrate the complexity of Hewison's suggestion, we might consider a scenario in which one member of a couple goes into a laborious description of outside events, while the other partner is rolling his eyes, strumming his fingers in impatience, and waiting for his turn. Even if the therapist can see the transitional phenomena in the description, how can he or she create an atmosphere in which the other partner can be enlisted to listen creatively and responsively to what seems to be, for him, lifeless speech? The therapist can try to find the developmental message in the speaking partner and invite the other partner's curiosity about it. However, as Hewison points out, there is always a danger of compliance and this approach can also potentially lead to a form of false self-compliance in the other partner, who may be trying to show the therapist that they are a good listener or a good patient.

## Trauma, psychic genera, and dissociation

Hewison introduces Bollas' (1992) concept of psychic genera to connect the idea of the couple making use of each other for developmental purposes with unconscious processes. Psychic genera are elements that link together unconscious aspects of experience, create new connections through association, and affect conscious experience. Psychic genera continue to accrue with experiences drawn in by the receptive unconscious which then organises similar experiences into constellations or clusters. "They become condensations of thousands of experiences and as we live and think, in time, our mind grows. The receptive unconscious stores unconscious perceptions, it organizes them, and it is the matrix of creativity" (Bollas, 2013, p. 28). Hewison says:

> We seek to make use of objects which are imbued with aspects of our unconscious through this process. These have entered the unconscious without being repressed because the unconscious is receptive; they have not been subject to symbolisation and so are "unthought knowns."
>
> (This volume, p. 7)

In a clinical example that demonstrates working in this model, Hewison described supervising a colleague to identify the "no-fly zone" for the man in a couple, rather than encouraging him to interpret a projective process. In this case, the technique was highly effective, because the therapist allowed something to emerge rather than interpreting it away. Hewison links this outcome to Bollas's theory of trauma because he sees trauma as inducing a need for protection, shutting down the receptive unconscious for making associations or gathering new experiences, and making sure nothing similar gets in again. For Hewison, networks of association are stunted, and nothingness is sought as respite from pain.

Hewison's emphasis on the retreat to nothingness overlaps with the deadening of experience associated with dissociation (Bromberg, 2003; Goldberg, 2017). In dissociation, the total state of the psyche/soma is in profound disconnection. The disconnection can be between psyche and soma, as well as, between the self and the external environment. In dissociated states, when significant trauma is a factor, the channels of communication between aspects of the psyche are cut off from clusters of associations, and the person can be so profoundly disconnected that they appear to be in an altered state of consciousness.

## Working with trauma in couples

Rather than a deadening of experience, we sometimes see heightened arousal and increased intensity of emotional experience when working with traumatised couples. In some cases, this heightened arousal may be a positive development that occurs when there is enough containment provided by the therapeutic setting. Some patients can experience the emotions connected to a trauma more vitally with their partner than they had when the original trauma occurred – as "apres coup," or "*Nachträglichkeit*" (Freud, 1966). In these instances, there has been enough maturation and safety with both the partner and the therapist to really experience the emotions of the traumatic event, perhaps for the first time.

In common parlance, people refer to being "triggered" and patients seem to understand well what this means. Something inside them, stemming from past traumatic experience, is being poked at by something in the present, perhaps by something in the behaviour of their partner. These triggered states can lead to intense fighting, failures to communicate, and a kind of deadlock. In these cases, when underlying trauma is at the root of the fighting, helping each partner to identify what is being "triggered" from the past trauma can take some of the pressure off and allow each of them to learn more about their partner's inner world. Often intense repetitive fights are the result of what I call "cross-triggers," when each partner is simultaneously poking at the other's trauma. These incidents require careful work by the couple therapist to allow room for these separate developmental bids within the fighting to be understood and this can be especially delicate and difficult when working with two traumatised partners in a couple.

## Conclusion

In an extremely meaningful way that is crucial to our work with couples, these ideas offer us a new language and a way of working that helps us to find the growth edge in the interactions, even in the most difficult sessions with couples. Hewison highlights how we must strive to find the creative edge even within the most maddening of repetitions. With this new understanding and its influence on our technique, we can attempt to create a facilitating environment that allows couples to create something new together, even when this type of interaction may appear, at first glance, to be destructive.

In conclusion, Hewison's contribution of treating creativity as primary provides a welcome addition and perspective to the psychoanalytic work with couples. In this discussion, I have elaborated Hewison's ideas and explored in depth what might be involved in incorporating "creativity as primary" in psychoanalytic couple psychotherapy. I have explored some initial ideas about what might be involved in cultivating creativity and imagination in ourselves and in our couples. Some key elements of this perspective include cultivating states of mind within ourselves, seeing subjective stories as creative perspectives to be worked with, and finding the creative edge in the repetitions that are inevitable in couples.

It is my hope that this model will offer couple therapists the courage and techniques to find the developmental and creative movement within all couples. It is within the safety of the couple relationship, and in the context of the containment provided by a good-enough couple psychotherapist, that couples can find new ways to foster communication, connection, and development. Couple psychotherapy, practised with these ideas in mind, can broaden the imagination and creative scope for both individuals in the relationship, separately and together.

## References

Arieti, S. (1976). *Creativity: The magic synthesis*. New York: Basic Books.
Bion, W. (1963). *Elements of psychoanalysis*. London: Routledge.
Bion, W. (1967). Notes on memory and desire. *The Psychoanalytic Forum*, 2(3), 271–280.
Bollas, C. (1992). *Being a character*. New York: Routledge.
Bollas, C. (2013). *The Freudian moment*. London: Karnac Books.
Breuer, J., & Freud, S. (1957). *Studies on hysteria*. New York: Basic Books.

Bromberg, P. M. (2003). Something wicked this way comes: Trauma, dissociation, and conflict: The space where psychoanalysis, cognitive science, and neuroscience overlap. *Psychoanalytic Psychology*, *20*(3), 558–574.

Freud, S. (1922). *Beyond the pleasure principle*. Trans. by C. J. M. Hubback. London: International Psycho-Analytical; Bartleby.com, 2010.

Freud, S. (1966). *Project for a scientific psychology* (1950 [1895]). United Kingdom: Hogarth Press.

Friend, J. (2013). Love as creative illusion and its place in psychoanalytic couple psychotherapy. *Couple and Family Psychoanalysis*, *3*(1), 3–14.

Goldberg, P. (2017). Fabricated Bodies: A Model for the Somatic False Self. *The International Journal of Psychoanalysis*, *85*(4), 823–840.

Grotstein, J. S. (2007). *A beam of intense darkness: Wilfred Bion's legacy to psychoanalysis*. London: Karnac.

Krist, E. (1952). *Psychoanalytic explorations in art*. New York: International Universities Press.

Morgan, M. (2001). First contacts: The therapist's "couple state of mind" as a factor in containment of couples seen for consultation. In F. Grier (Ed.), *Brief encounters with couples* (pp. 17–32). London: Karnac.

Nettleton, S. (2017). *The metapsychology of Christopher Bollas: An introduction*. New York: Routledge.

Ogden, T. H. (2005). *Reverie and interpretation: Sensing something human*. London: Karnac Books.

Winnicott, D. W. (1953). Transitional objects and transitional phenomena – a study of the first not-me possession. *International Journal of Psychoanalysis*, *34*, 89–97.

Winnicott, D. W. (1965). Ego distortion in terms of true and false self. In *The maturational process and the facilitating environment: Studies in the theory of emotional development* (pp. 140–157). New York: International Universities Press, Inc.

Winnicott, D. W. (1971). *Playing and reality*. Oxford: Penguin.

Winnicott, D. W. (1973). *The child, the family, and the outside world*. Oxford: Penguin.

# Chapter 3

# Love as creative illusion and its place in psychoanalytic couple psychotherapy[1]

*Julie Friend*

Lisa and John entered my office some years ago, bringing with them an unusually pressured, urgent atmosphere. Lisa, reed-thin and intense, let me know at the start that we had three weeks. She would not wait any longer for John to decide whether or not they were getting married – she had set a deadline, and she would not humiliate herself further by going one day beyond it. I learned from the monologue she delivered through clenched teeth that they had in fact had a wedding planned one year ago. Everything had been set to go, and John pulled out of that plan several days before they were to have been married. She was completely humiliated that she was still waiting – that he could still not decide. John sat, baseball hat on his head, good-looking and silent, his jaw muscles tense as he chewed gum and for quite some time said nothing. He seemed cold, or anxious, maybe both – I couldn't tell. Nor could I read the impact Lisa's demands and upset had on him at first, but he gradually spoke of his concerns about, what he perceived, as her eating disorder, and his worries about her lack of acceptance of his family's religious observances.

There was a great deal to think about quickly with Lisa and John. I wondered about the meanings of the pressured atmosphere of their relationship, about the separation issues from their families of origin, and about the split with which they divided their feelings about their relationship, with John ostensibly carrying all of the ambivalence and anxiety about marriage, and Amy all of the urgent desire and demand. I wondered about her eating disorder, his silence, and the sadomasochistic gridlock (Morgan, 1995) of their engagement. It seemed to me that John's need to keep their relationship from moving forward might

1 This chapter is dedicated to the memory of James Fisher, the depth and richness of whose warm thinking has been such an inspiration to me and many of my colleagues.

DOI: 10.4324/9781003265023-3

mirror Lisa's need to keep her weight exactly where it was; what was this need for control about? John's refusal to move ahead clearly intensified Lisa's anxiety, which, in turn, intensified John's fears of marrying her. On a practical level, I wondered how to help them open up a space to think in the face of the three-week deadline Lisa had announced, and whether it would be possible to help them at all. What, indeed, would help even consist of?

As I was thinking about these dynamics between them, Lisa sharply asked John if he was staying with her only out of responsibility, guilty about his wish to leave her. The demand and anger in her tone was underpinned with poignant fear. With genuine emotion in his voice, John's face darkened, and he told her no. He said he did feel guilty, but about not marrying her and also not *leaving* her, so that she could be free to move on. He didn't want to leave her, but he didn't understand what was holding him back, and didn't know if he would be able to figure it out. He worried he was being unfair to her and selfish.

Lisa began to cry. She said,

> I don't know what to do! I love John, I love him so much – if I thought he would really be happier without me, it would be awful, it would break my heart, but I would go. But I think he is so unhappy! And he loves me, I know he does, I think he is stuck in something with his family, and I am so worried that if I leave, he will be stuck all his life, and miserable, and that just breaks my heart! I'm afraid he will never be happy; I want to pull him out of it. I know he loves me; I know we can be happy together, but he is stuck in something! And I can't wait forever; I don't know what to do!

With that I felt dropped down with a thump into a different register. My attention was taken almost entirely by the intensity of what my body was feeling. My heart was pounding hard and ached in my chest, and for quite a few minutes it took a significant effort to hold back my tears. I was shocked and overwhelmed by how deeply moved I felt by this couple I had met minutes ago and thought: "They *love* each other! I have to DO something!" and then wondered what on earth that even meant. I reminded myself that I was in the grip of a powerful countertransference reaction, and that Lisa and John had been unusually effective in quickly bringing me into their world. Yet these thoughts, while accurate and containing, had a defensive quality as well, and seemed to be an effort at minimising the emotional and intensely embodied elements of an experience that I found powerfully compelling, destabilising, and confusing. The otherwise rich, complex body of theory in the psychoanalytic literature on couples in which I root my work surprisingly does not say much about love and didn't seem to address something elemental to the experience with Lisa and John.

This chapter is an attempt to explore a paradox. Psychoanalytic couple psychotherapy emphasises building depressive position capacities, aiming to help couples to think more clearly about each other, and strengthen their ability to perceive each other more realistically. And yet love, at the very heart of couple relationships, is a state that is often far from realistic – it can be full of idealisation, blurred boundaries, fantasy, and illusion. Is there a place in psychoanalytic psychotherapy with couples for listening on a separate register to the intense, non-reasonable emotional vicissitudes of love? Is it useful to consider balancing the emphasis on the value of mature, realistic relating with that of less rational, more embodied forms of relating in couples? How do we as couple psychotherapists hold a place for both, and help couples build their capacity to hold a tension between more mature, reasoned kinds of relating on the one hand, with the creative potential of less rational, more aesthetic qualities of relating on the other?

Following my encounter with Lisa and John, I asked many colleagues whether they think about love when they are working with couples, curious to know how they struggle with these questions. Almost all of them looked surprised at the question, and to *my* surprise many answered, "No, not really." While clinically intense states of love can often tend to be minimised or viewed in pathological terms, I am proposing the alternative idea that romantic and passionate love is a major arena in which we experience a creative engagement with the world. I will consider love as a creative illusion: the beloved is, in some measure, both a part of oneself and a separate other, occupying in Alvarez' words, "an intermediate area of experience in between pure narcissistic illusion that everything belongs to oneself and the mature awareness of separateness and indebtedness, where true symbolic functioning is possible" (Alvarez, 1996, p. 377).

Approaching love as an inherently creative psychic state rich with developmental potential, I will suggest that attention to such emotionally intense currents within couple relationships should have a more considered place in psychoanalytic couple psychotherapy. I will also discuss some clinical implications of these ideas.

The powerful emotions in the room with Lisa and John directed my attention towards taking a different perspective from the one with which I ordinarily thought about and organised my work with a couple. Another response I got from colleagues with whom I spoke about this session was, "What do you mean by *love*?" That's certainly a good question – how *do* we talk about love? In English, the word love can refer to many different emotional experiences: affection, attraction, lust, care, passion, regard, infatuation, worship, possession, and affinity, to mention a few. We use the word love not only in relation to our romantic attachments, but also in describing feelings for our friends, children, parents, our work, a movie, a favourite flavour of ice cream… Thinking about the subject of love in terms of couple relating is further complicated, as love is mercurial, transient, unruly, always mixed with other emotions such as dependency, and is usually mixed with some measure of aggression. It is unpredictable, uncontrollable, and sometimes uncontainable. It takes many forms—passionate, possessive, kind, concerned, filial, destructive—and its forms can change and blur.

I searched the literature on psychoanalytic psychotherapy with couples. Love is not explored systematically there as a clinical entity, neither in terms of what seems to be felt or not felt by the couple, nor in terms of the ways the therapist's perception of the presence or absence of love in the couple impacts on the clinical field. In his scholarly exploration of tensions inherent in couple relating, Fisher (1999) contrasts what he calls "marriage," which he defines as "the passion for and dependence on the intimate other" (ibid, p. 1) with narcissism, "a longing for an other that is perfectly attuned … and thus not a genuine other at all" (ibid, pp. 1–2). While Fisher describes marriage as "perhaps the most complex and difficult encounter with the beauty of the object," referring also to "passionate intimacy with another human being" (ibid, p. 11); notably, he does not call this encounter love (Fisher, 1999). The absence of love in the literature is particularly curious, and paradoxical, since we would all probably agree that most couple relationships begin within some experience of, or hope of, love. Love is at the core of the western view of couple relationships, and it is frequently a feeling of loss of love, or trouble with love, that brings couples to us for help.

There is an implicit assumption throughout the literature that build-ing healthy couple relating always involves a strengthened relationship with reality, including the capacity to bear disappointment, and what is generally referred to as disillusionment. We try to help couples see each other clearly and realistically. Couples are best equipped to weather the strains and changes in life if they can bear to mourn what is not possible, what has been lost, or what must be given up. All of this is in keeping with the task of encouraging and building capacities that are related to depressive position functioning: the softening of omnipotence, the capacity to mourn, and the ability to feel genuine concern and empathy for a separate other.

When love is directly mentioned in the psychoanalytic couple liter-ature, it is generally viewed like other experiences of strong emotion, as potentially growth-promoting, provided the couple has the capacity to think about and process intensely felt experiences between them. Love tends to be seen as something best abided in a reasonable and realistic form. Morgan, for example, in *On Being Able to Be a Couple*, states:

> it is of course quite common for couples to seek and aspire to a merged state of mind, feeling this to be the essence of being in love. However, *true and sustaining love* [my italics] comes only with the disillusionment of this idea of merger as the ideal.
>
> (Morgan, 2005, p. 28)

Privileging mature and differentiated relating, she goes on to suggest that:

> Once the couple has given up the idea of merger as the ideal that they have to strive for, it becomes more possible from time to time to move into that state spontaneously, for example during sex, and to enjoy the intense feeling it arouses; and it is also more possible to move out of it again, without too much regret.
>
> (Morgan, 2005, p. 28)

This sounds like a very reasonable and sensible balance, but love can be unruly and is often not reasonable at all. States of powerful love don't exactly fit into this template. Is it our aim for couples to be rea-sonably passionate? If so, what is sacrificed in attaining this goal?

"What is love?" – a complicated question indeed. While I think about love quite a lot in my work, and it is something that I tend to try to track with couples, it is very difficult to think about in a clear or systematic way, or to describe. The stories couples tell about their initial meeting and the beginning of their relationship have always seemed to me to be of privileged importance, showing a dream they had had about their relationship, about who they were, and who and what they were hoping for. In his essay *On First Impressions*, as re-produced in *The Apprehension of Beauty*, Meltzer describes "the phenomenon of … love [as] founded upon a primal dream of love" which "entitles [love] to enlistment in the general phenomenology of the transference" (Meltzer, 1988, p. 38). Notably, this is very different from a love that is realistic, and has weathered disillusionment. He goes on to quote Robert Louis Stevenson:

> Two persons, neither of them, it may be, very amiable or very beautiful, meet, speak a little, and look a little into each other's eyes. That has been done a dozen or so times in the experience of either with no great result. But on this occasion all is different. They fall at once into that state in which another person becomes to us the very gist and centre-point of God's creation…and the love of life itself is translated into a wish to remain in the same world with so precious and desirable a fellow creature.
>
> (Stevenson, 1881, p. 11)

Such transporting, transformative encounters may be enviable, but they are not primarily realistic. Experiences of love cannot be accounted for in terms of depressive position functioning alone. The two people in a moment such as this don't actually know each other; their meeting is fuelled by attraction, need, and large measures of illusion, imagination, idealisation, and projection. Milner states that:

> to find the familiar in the unfamiliar require(s) an ability to tolerate the temporary loss of the sense of self … it perhaps requires a state of mind which has been described by Berensen (1950) as "the aesthetic moment" … the two become one entity; time and space are abolished and (they are) possessed by one awareness.
>
> (Milner, 1952, p. 189)

All goodness, all of the promise of life, is suddenly represented by, embodied by, the beloved other. Intense romantic love has as a central quality, at least some of the time, a blurring of self and other. This can be experienced as an intense need to be as near as possible to the beloved, and an equally intense fear of losing them. In these urgent longings, and in the powerful feeling that one has met someone one already knew, or was waiting for, there is a large measure of what we would, in other circumstances, see as unrealistic or magical thinking.

Those who have written about love in psychoanalysis, (Bergmann, 1987; Green and Kohon, 2005; Person, 1988) note that it is a topic usually left for the realms of poetry, music, and art. Person observes that psychoanalysis, like "most academic disciplines either ignore[s] love or treat[s] it in accordance with the rationalist tradition" (Person, 1988, p. 16). She points out that,

> rationalists counsel a cool approach (and) ...distinguish "mature" love from romantic love...Their hope is that tamed, mutual love will be less disorderly than romantic love.... Romantics, on the other hand, see the rationalist view as love with the heart cut out.
>
> (Person, 1988, p. 17)

In psychoanalysis as a whole, Person observes that love tends to be framed in terms of its "mature" iterations.

A good example of this is Kernberg's cataloguing of types of love as mature or pathological. He maps out the complexity of interweaving elements that are involved in sustaining what he views as mature sexual love. Kernberg sees being in love (rather than falling in love) as a complex achievement that involves many different elements: sexual excitement transformed into sexual desire for the other; tenderness that results from the integration of libidinally and aggressively invested self and object representations, with love predominating over aggression; an ability to tolerate normal ambivalence; an ability to identify with the partner, including reciprocal gender identification; what he interestingly calls "mature idealisation" along with a deep commitment to the other and to the relationship; and lastly, "the passionate character of the love relation in all three aspects: the sexual relationship, object relationship and the superego investment of the couple" (Kernberg, 1995, p. 32).

Kernberg's delineation of what a monumental and complex psychological task it is to maintain a loving couple relationship is impressive and useful. It clarifies what a layered and complex job we have in helping couples develop a relationship that can weather time, and change, and stay emotionally alive. Kernberg's work, however, is also an excellent example of approaching love from a rationalist perspective. André Green, in *Love and Its Vicissitudes*, notes that "the psychoanalytic view (of love) misses something which is lost in its description of love" (Green and Kohon, 2005, p. 5).

My experience with John and Lisa brought this "something," the emotional life or tone between a couple, the presence or absence of a feeling of love, to the foreground for me. It was a turning point, and my attention was taken for some time on trying to track my sense of the emotional connections in the couples with whom I was working, and also some sense of how my relation to them and to the work was affected by what I perceived in this arena. It is a skewed sample, certainly – couples who come in for help are struggling, and that usually, but not always, affects how they feel about one another. Over time, I have found that in some way the couple relationship seems less hopeful, more concerning to me when it is characterised by cool indifference. I am generally more optimistic even with couples who are highly reactive to one another, sensing that there is some way they affect each other and need one another. This is important to note, because some of the more heated couples really can have quite a difficult time hearing each other and working together, elements ordinarily considered hallmarks of healthy couple functioning.

I would not want to suggest, however, that a couple's feeling of love for one another always bodes well. It is important to consider distinctions between a couple's capacity for passion along with other factors that affect the viability of the relationship. It is true they must have some ability to think about their emotional experience of each other. In addition, as with any other quality of relating, there is of course a wide range of what sort of emotional atmosphere works for different couples, what they feel most at home with.

That said, I do look for sparks to orient my work with couples. Some couples talk quite a bit about their passionate connection and their love and desire for one another, or display it, talking a great deal about their passionate sexual connection, for example. It is sometimes easy to pathologise those couples, who can seem overly wild about each other, in terms of the intensity of their needs for merger, or what we could see as a predominance of dependence between them. And there are couples whose every move or word triggers an avalanche of mutual overreaction that they *call* love, while all we see is dependency, sado-masochism, desperation, and a furious cycle of mutual projection. Other couples can appear mature, realistic, and caring and yet they may be living in a spare emotional atmosphere. They may have a very strong capacity to see one another as separate, and communicate well, but experience little joy or passion or emotional connection with one another.

Another couple I saw some years ago brought the impact of a lack of a creative experience of love to my attention. Carol and Ed grew up in neighbouring towns on the East coast. Ed is steady, hard-working, and loyal. Carol is "wired," driven, and the only woman Ed has been with. Ed had been relieved to have been chosen, to have a girl and settle down into a good and safe life together. Carol, on the other hand, had felt Ed would be a "good husband; he was so nice," and as we talked further, it emerged that she had also been fleeing from a part of herself, a wild sexual self that was drawn to rough, not-so-nice, "bad boys."

They didn't present a pretty picture, really a pretty discouraging one. Carol was initially mean and provocative with Ed, bored and frustrated at home now that their son had gone off to college. It was generally very hard for Ed to begin to identify his emotions and to speak up directly about his experience with Carol in the marriage. He tended to feel wronged, stomped on, and often, for what we might see as good reason. Carol, for example, had had affairs, which he hated and was shamed by, but seemed to feel he had no choice but to tolerate. I imagined he was very afraid of his anger, determined not to be anything like a "bad boy" himself. I really wondered why they continued to stay together and thought of them as a "not-love" couple, because I couldn't see any sign of creative, generative engagement between them.

Yet Carol wanted to stay. She said wanted more contact with Ed. She felt lonely and isolated. While her considerable narcissism was a noteworthy element – she felt he never understood her quite correctly – her loneliness and despair were nonetheless palpable and affecting. Ed was indeed very controlled and hard to make any emotional contact with. I could see that Carol couldn't find any point of imaginative contact with Ed. She read his self-protectiveness as disinterest, and then provoked him more, in part in an effort to get some emotional response. Ed, of course, then retreated from her attacks on him. It felt terribly discouraging to be with them, and my experience was of working laboriously to reach out to each of them.

Then something happened that surprised me: one session Carol told us that she had had a dream of being in a house with a view of Paris, a beautiful house filled with light. As Ed and I looked puzzled about why she was telling us this dream, she turned to him, a bright (and unusual) smile appearing on her face and said to him "YOU were THERE in the house! I want YOU to be there!" I was surprised to hear this, and thought it might represent a wish on Carol's part for an adventurous, romantic connection with Ed. Ed, however, was bland in his reaction. I thought, or hoped, this might be an expression of a combination of surprise, his inexperience with emotion, self-protectiveness, and retaliation for ways Carol had hurt him. However, when I raised questions about his flat reaction to her dream, they both told me that this is how it has always been between them. This sort of "relating" felt comfortable and normal to Ed; painfully isolating to Carol.

It was one of those awful moments to witness with a couple. The hope represented by Carol's dream was shattered; her shoulders and face fell with disappointment and defeat after Ed's reaction. Carol was even more convinced than before that she and Ed could not meet in an emotionally engaged way. No longer having affairs, she was painfully certain she would have to go through life without ever feeling really alive or connected to him. Yet she saw he was a good guy, liked him, and wanted to stay married. It was a dark moment. I could hear no dream of transporting, transformative engagement with one another, nor any hope of creative possibility. Soon after, they decided to move back East where Ed had a job offer and where they would be closer to their families.

It seemed to me that Carol and Ed's relationship was extremely impoverished, because they did not share a way to meet emotionally, and this led me to consider love from the perspective of transitional and aesthetic phenomena. The transitional object represents a paradox, an intermediate area of experience between the inner and outer worlds. This back and forth between inside and outside continues to be important and vitalising, all through life. The interpenetration of *different* levels of reality, both objective and subjective, is a crucial element in the experience of creativity and liveliness. In addressing such experiences, Bollas describes the aesthetic moment as carrying an "illusion of deep rapport between subject and object" (Bollas, 1978, p. 385) The aesthetic moment holds transformational potential, as it promises an experience "where the unintegrations of self find integrations through the form provided by the transformational object" (ibid, p. 385). Carol and Ed could not "find" each other, or allow for the degree of merger and of un-integration that I am proposing is an element of love.

Modell saw in Winnicott's idea of the transitional object "a testimony to the synthetic powers of Eros" (Modell, 1970, p. 243). Thinking of love as a sort of transitional experience is one way to account for both the creative exaltation in love, and for the deadness when it is absent, when there is no shared psychological world in which the partners are living. Viewed through this lens, the loved object is *both* real and created, and then, in turn, also has an impact on the creation of the sense of self. A strange and magical alchemy can happen in love – one both finds what or who one imagined, outside of oneself, and at the same time, one's sense of oneself is transformed by the encounter with the other.

André Green states that "ultimately the experience of love teaches us that it is linked to illusion" (Green and Kohon, 2005, p. 16). There is an important distinction to consider between illusion and idealisation. Idealisation is an element of falling in love, and as we learn more about our partner, and they become more "real" to us, less "a bundle of projections" (Winnicott, 1969, p. 712). It is inevitable that some of the idealisation must fade, and we must mourn its loss. In contrast, disillusionment means something more problematic, a potential threat to a creative relation inside oneself to one's partner. Illusion is indispensable as a form of vitalising engagement with life, and it is often through an experience of love and merger with another that it is refreshed and re-created. Meltzer was mindful of this element of ambiguity between the partner we imagine and the actual other, the interplay between internal and external, when he said:

> ... our minds are full of characters in search ... of players to fit the parts. Thus, does transference people the intimate area of our lives. If we go on learning from experience the drama changes and

may require recasting. If we are neurotic, the drama remains fixed, and may require recasting as the actors grow jaded by the parts imposed upon them. With rare good luck the growing person finds like growth in his players and they write and play the new dramas together. With rare bad luck the neurotic finds his players never tire of their roles and they proceed through life in an interminable "mousetrap."

(Meltzer, 1988, p. 470)

Thinking of love as a creative illusion has direct clinical implications. We do need to help couples traverse necessary and inevitable de-idealisation as they go through life together. It is useful, and important, that they are able to face the truth of who they each are. It is important for them to see their real strengths and weaknesses, both to build an experience of intimacy and to be known in a way that feels real. They can also thus construct a relationship in which they know what they can and cannot expect from one another. The loss of idealisation can be replaced, in part, with the pleasure and interest in getting to know a partner more fully, and in being known more deeply ourselves.

Yet it is also important to watch for disillusionment and to think carefully about what we are seeing, since this can be a more malignant and destructive experience. My concerns are raised by couples who don't seem to meet in a "transitional realm" in which they can experience an enriching back and forth between their senses of internal and external reality (Winnicott, 1953) when one or both seem truly indifferent to the other, even politely so. Their prospects seem much more hopeful when there is a sense of a shared connection, even if it appears fraught.

If we consider love as a kind of transitional experience, perhaps there are also times in any couple relationship when it is necessary to leave things unsaid, and unknown, to leave room for what is imagined in each partner about the other. Perhaps that is just possible when things are going well and creatively between partners. Of course, for love to be sustained, it must include relating to the other as a whole and separate object. At the same time, the importance of preserving some degree of a more non-realistic, aesthetic investment in the other has been underrepresented in psychoanalytic thinking about couples.

I'd like to consider for a moment why this might be. Certainly, one element might be the continuing legacy of the conflict between the rationalist and romantic traditions. This is evident in the emphasis on *thinking* in the psychoanalytic literature on couple psychotherapy. Yet in our current day, when the multiplicity of experience is widely accepted, the absence in the literature of a more considered place for love is noteworthy. Perhaps the presence of loving experiences of love in our consulting rooms can be problematic for us. Depending on the state of our own private lives, we might feel envious of love in couples we see. Witnessing these states may also raise many kinds of Oedipal anxieties about intruding, being excluded, peeking, and the like. All of these could lead us to defensively disparage or minimise love when we do see it. I have noticed that I tend automatically to avert my eyes during moments of certain warmth, or playful tenderness, or a sexual current in a couple interaction. I can feel awkward being in the room with them at such times, as if I am transgressing: what am I DOING there? And what is it we SHOULD do, what is our task, with a couple who are engaged with each other in an aesthetic way?

In spite of our awkwardness, love from the perspective of transitional and aesthetic phenomena deserves further theoretical exploration. Although complicated by questions of definition and subjectivity, love is of particular importance when we consider the enriching and developmental possibilities that less-differentiated forms of relating can offer. In our clinical work, I propose that we approach love and its ebb and flow between couples as an additional axis along which to think about the couple relationship, holding a space in our minds for its creative possibilities. It is precisely the ambiguous, imagined aspects of the experience of the other that can fuel a rich, revitalising, and creative potential in each member of the couple. We can see it sometimes in glances exchanged; a smile of delight; concentration when listening to the other talk about something that is difficult to hear; in a look of tender compassion; or when hands entwine. Whether we respond with silence or with playful engagement, these are important observations that warrant our thoughtful attention.

## References

Alvarez, A. (1996). The clinician's debt to Winnicott. *Journal of Child Psychotherapy*, 22, 377–383.

Bergmann, M. S. (1987). *The anatomy of loving*. New York: Columbia University Press.

Bollas, C. (1978). The aesthetic moment and the search for transformation. *The Annual of Psychoanalysis*, 6, 385–394.

Fisher, J. V. (1999). *The uninvited guest*. London: Karnac.

Green, A., & Kohon, G. (2005). *Love and its vicissitudes*. London: Routledge Press.

Kernberg, O. (1995). *Love relations, normality and pathology*. New Haven: Yale University Press.

Meltzer, D. (1988). *The apprehension of beauty*. Scotland: Clunie Press. Reprinted 2004, London: Karnac & the Meltzer Harris Trust.

Milner, M. (1952). Aspects of symbolism in comprehension of the not-self. *International Journal of Psycho-Analysis*, 33, 181–194.

Modell, A. H. (1970). The transitional object and the creative act. *Psychoanalytic Quarterly*, 39, 240–250.

Morgan, M. (1995). The projective gridlock: A form of identification in couple relationships. In: S. Ruszczynski & J. Fisher (Eds.), *Intrusiveness and intimacy in the couple* (pp. 33–48). London: Karnac.

Morgan, M. (2005). On being able to be a couple: The importance of a "creative couple" in psychic life. In: F. Grier (Ed.), *Oedipus and the couple* (pp. 9–30). London: Karnac.

Person, E. S. (1988). *Dreams of love and fateful encounters*. New York: Penguin Books.

Stevenson, R. L. S. (1881). *Virginibus puerisque & other papers*.

Winnicott, D. W. (1953). Transitional objects and transitional phenomena—a study of the first not-me possession. *International Journal of Psychoanalysis*, 34, 89–97.

Winnicott, D. W. (1969). The use of an object. *International Journal of Psycho-Analysis*, 50, 711–716.

# Chapter 4

# Discussion of "Love as creative illusion and its place in psychoanalytic couple psychotherapy"

*Rachael Peltz*

I will begin this discussion with a quote from Adam Phillips:

> Lovers, of course, are notoriously frantic epistemologists, second only to paranoiacs (and analysts) as readers of signs and wonders. But what would falling in love look like if knowledge of oneself or another, of oneself as another, was not the aim or result? What would we be doing together if we were not getting to know each other? Another way of saying this might be to imagine a meeting or a relationship without (answerable) questions … "How do I know if I know someone?" is a very different question from "How do I know if I love or desire someone?" Some people would never have known if they had never heard of knowing
>
> (Phillips, 1994, p. 41)

In Phillips's typically vexing manner, he asks, "How do I know if I love or desire someone? Some people would never know if they had never heard of knowing," suggesting that the felt experience of loving and knowing live in very different registers. In this chapter, Julie Friend joins Philips by directing the reader to these different registers: the registers of loving on the one hand and knowing on the other – and how we may address these separate registers in our clinical work with couples.

In his book, *On Flirtation* (1994), Phillips recommends that we analysts and clinicians "flirt" with ideas generated inside and outside of the corpus of psychoanalytic theorising, rather than being – in his words, "stifled" by the ways in which "psychoanalytic writing has become a way of making or joining clubs" (p. xi). "Flirtation" he writes, "keeps things in play, and by doing so lets us get to know them in different ways" (p. xii). In her paper, Friend does more than flirt with

DOI: 10.4324/9781003265023-4

ideas at the margins of the Tavistock tradition in which she received her psychoanalytic couples training. She uses the fullness of her own experience as a couple psychotherapist as a window into attending to questions about the felt experience of "love." She marvels at how little love is referred to in the analytic couple literature and highlights Person's (1988) observation that psychoanalysis, like "most academic disciplines either ignore[s] love or treat[s] it in accordance with the rationalist tradition" (Friend, this volume, p. 39). In accordance with her desire to enrich and expand how we think about love and couples work, Friend "keeps things in play" by reaching to Winnicott, and other analytic voices in the Independent Tradition, to get to know couples and the love between them in evocatively new ways.

Friend asks a series of questions in the opening of her paper:

> … Is there a place in psychoanalytic psychotherapy with couples for *listening on a separate register* to the intense, non-reasonable emotional vicissitudes of love? Is it useful to consider balancing the emphasis on the value of mature, realistic relating with that of less rational, more embodied forms of relating in couples? How do couple therapists hold a place for both, and help couples build their capacity to hold a tension between more mature, reasoned kinds of relating on the one hand, with the creative potential of less rational, more aesthetic qualities of relating on the other?
>
> (p. 35 italics added)

To address these questions, I will concentrate on this *separate register* to which Friend refers. I will also follow Friend's lead in positioning this separate register within the paradoxical sensibility of Winnicott's developmental schema, such that love becomes, as an outgrowth of Friend's flirtation with Winnicott's ideas, a form of "creative illusion." I will also consider how this way of thinking can help our clinical work with couples.

## The embodied, visceral register of being (in love)

Friend begins her paper by introducing us to Lisa and John, a couple polarised in the midst of deciding about the future of their relationship and whether or not to marry. After Lisa issues a compassionate testimonial of her dilemma, one that registers as resoundingly true to Friend, she notes that she felt "dropped down with a thump into a different register" (p. 34). Her heart was pounding hard and ached in her chest and she worked to hold back tears. Compelled by Lisa's heartfelt plea, Friend thought, "They love each other! I have to do something!" (p. 34). Presumably, her thought was to attend to the stalemate between them, while helping this couple salvage their love. Lisa and John were able to successfully convey the desperate state of their life together, a state in which the stakes were very high. To my ear, Friend entered a visceral, even primal, register when she "dropped down with a thump." Something deeply precious and powerful was at risk (of dying, being lost, or no longer being). Feeling this, Friend thought to herself, "I have to do something!", as if to imagine throwing a life preserver to this drowning couple and pulling them to solid ground – the ground of Being, upon which one must be firmly planted in order to hope, to "know," or discover anything. And sometimes we must "do" things in our clinical work that are more significant than anything we could meaningfully "say." The "life" of this couple was at stake. Because of her sensitivity and receptivity to her own internal state of mind and body, Friend was able to enter this visceral register. Then, sensing the risk of starvation in the couple, Friend reached to theory and began her investigation into the literature on love.

It is no accident that references to love are not often seen in the analytic literature. Our theories have largely addressed the epistemological domain to which Philips refers. Psychoanalytic theory has largely addressed the domain of meaning; the search for understanding; the cultivation of the capacity to meaningfully inquire and thereby "know" things about ourselves and the unconscious forces at play, and the question of what mental states we are in when we can or can't think in order to discover and know things. With these aims in mind, clinical work with individuals and couples (and groups) has emphasised strengthening our reflective, representational capacities. However, Friend seems to be directing us to a different register, *not as a substitute by any means*, but rather as an embodied visceral, more implicit counterpoint – one that we may think of as intuitive, procedural, and often out of our awareness. In her effort to listen in a different register, I read Friend as searching for a way to describe and delineate the subjective resonances one can experience in the company of couples – one that resides more in depth than in the general category of countertransference. I read her as reaching for, what I think of, as the "ground" of contact-making.

I have written elsewhere (Peltz, 2018, 2021) about the growing literature addressing the "ground" level of clinical work that is based on the synthesis of theories coming from many directions – including infant-parent research; developmental and child analytic work (especially with severely disturbed children on the autistic-psychotic spectrum; intersubjective and Bionian field theories; unrepresented states; trauma theory; and more. This literature attends to the non-representational, procedural, and embodied dimensions of our clinical work in which we strive to acutely sense and reach toward active engagement, and adjust what and how we communicate in order to join our patients where "they are," and sometimes attempt to pull them out of dangerously undrawn, death-like states (Alvarez, 2012; Durbin, 2014). In this way, we are reaching to engage our patients *in being with us* by actively being, and sometimes *doing*, with them. This is a different register – *a pre-reflective, somato-psychic, experiencing register of being and being with* (Eshel, 2013). This points to ways of theorising the "contacting" dimension of our work that goes beyond privileging the capacity to symbolise, which is the hallmark of more typical "interpretive" interventions (Peltz, 2018, p. 362). This visceral contact-making register is one we all share; one that we all need to be spoken to and engaged with in a manner that makes visceral sense to us. Winnicott (1964) reminded us that

> in each baby is a *vital spark* and this urge toward life and growth and development is part of the baby, something the child is born with and which is carried forward in a way that we do not have to understand.
>
> (p. 27)

I think Friend is suggesting that when the vital spark and urge toward life that is present in all of us is ignited with another person, this experience forms the ground of being in love. This is something one senses is present (or not) in the company of couples. Indeed, she references "look[ing] for sparks to orient [her]work with couples" (this volume, p. 40).

In a recent paper, summarising these shifts in thinking in psychoanalysis, Ogden (2019) discusses the differences between what he calls,

> … epistemological psychoanalysis (having to do with knowing and understanding) for which Freud and Klein are principal authors, and ontological psychoanalysis (having to do with being and becoming), for which Winnicott and Bion are principal architects).
>
> (p. 661)

One could say that ontological psychoanalysis addresses the experiencing realm of being and forms the ground for later discoveries of representational meanings, which in the language of Bion (1970), translates into the movement from "O" into "K." We constantly move between these realms in our clinical work, and it is in this capacity Friend is enriching the domain of couple therapy.

In her paper, Friend offers another clinical vignette from the therapy of Carol and Ed. She calls them a "not love" couple because she "could not see any sign of creative, generative engagement between them" (this volume, p. 41). Carol felt lonely and isolated: "She never felt he understood her quite correctly." Ed, in turn felt: "wronged, stomped on, and, often, for what we might see as good reason" (this volume, p. 41). Friend described an hour in which Carol shared a dream of being in a beautiful, light-filled house with a view of Paris, and she exuberantly exclaimed that, in the dream, Ed was *there* (with her) in the house! "I want *you* to be there!", she said. Sadly, Ed seemed not to register the significance of this dream for Carol, nor did it elicit any curiosity or emotion in him. When Friend inquired about the flatness of his response, the couple remarked that exchanges like this were the order of the day. "This sort of 'relating' felt comfortable and normal to Ed; (and) painfully isolating to Carol" (this volume, p. 42).

No doubt there are many couples like Carol and Ed who arrive in our offices feeling misunderstood, dejected, and alone, engendering sadness in the ways that Friend describes. Each member feels unseen in essential ways – that is, in the ways they feel most *alive as who they are*. Both feel each other's "vital spark" to be doused by the other. Like Friend, I have witnessed many couples who feel "you don't get me" in response to their partners.

To better understand what was happening (or not happening) between Lisa and John, and Carol and Ed, Friend turns to Winnicott's (1971) paradoxical developmental schema, notably his conception of transitional objects and phenomena. Here, Friend finds what she is looking for: a model that describes the process of creative engagement underlying our most intense and meaningful emotional attachments, including our romantic and loving partnerships. For Winnicott, development itself is an inherently creative process, in so far as each step of the way a person puts their personal stamp on the stuff of life presented before her/him. The play between imagination and externality is always in motion. if all goes well (enough). This puts a new cast on the question of "reality" and perception. To the extent that Klein (1930) devised the epistemophilic drive as a primary urge *to know*, Winnicott designates "Primary creativity *(as)* the form of non-defensive omnipotence that underpins vitality and makes reality 'feel real'" (Goldman, in press). Primary creativity then becomes the *throughline* in all Winnicott's ideas. Goldman continues:

> Winnicott ... shared with the Romantic poets a belief in what Coleridge referred to as Primary Imagination and Winnicott called primary creativity: psychic life is imbued with a form of non-defensive omnipotence that underpins vitality. Reality is not passively imprinted upon us but imaginatively elaborated from within us. The mind knows objects not by passive reception but by the vigor of its imaginative energy that empowers and authenticates perception granting meaning to brute facts. "When I look at the clock ...", Winnicott ... once remarked, "I create a clock, but I am careful not to see clocks except just where I already know there is one ..." Like the Romantic poets, Winnicott was less interested in "reality testing" than in how an individual's sense of reality is generated in the to-and-fro movement between imaginative apperception and objective perception .... "The fact is," Winnicott ... said, "that what we create is already there, but the creativeness lies in the way we get at perception through conception and apperception."
>
> (Goldman, in press)

As a complement to the wish to *understand* the couples she sees clinically, Friend suggests we consider the role of the presence (or absence) of the vital urge to (reciprocally and) non-defensively *create* our romantic partnerships. Like the mother of the child discovering the transitional object, the clinician must be present and allow creative imagination to flourish in the couple. In Winnicott's (1971) words:

> ... *it is a matter of agreement between us and the baby that we will never ask the question: Did you conceive of this or was it presented to you from without?" The important point is that no decision on this point is expected. The question is not to be formulated.*
>
> (p. 12, italics in original)

Couples for whom this fundamental question isn't asked – whether they created or found each other – are allowed the spontaneous (pro-cedural) movement necessary to "Be" and to continue "Becoming."

When this implicit understanding isn't present, one has the impres-sion of "endless processing" that comes to no avail. Such processing can erupt into an explosive battleground generating intransigent impasse (Goldner, 2017; Peltz, 2017), projective gridlock (Morgan, 1995), or lifeless stalemate akin to Carol and Ed. And we may encoun-ter couples somewhere in the middle of these two poles (Morgan, 2005) in which, like Lisa and John, they need *active* help unlocking the door to their creative and loving potential as a couple.

Returning to transitional objects and phenomena, Winnicott (1971) describes the:

> ... intermediate state of experiencing, to which inner reality and external life both contribute. It is an area that is not challenged, because no claim is made on its behalf except that it shall exist as a resting-place for the individual engaged in the perpetual human task of keeping inner and outer reality separated yet interrelated.
>
> (p. 2)

In turning our attention to love as a creative illusion and its place in couple psychotherapy, Friend directs us to consider that the capacity to hold this paradoxical tension exists as a foundational resting place – a ground of being – for couples, in that they have both found and created each other. In our work with couples, we may ask ourselves, along with Friend and Winnicott (1971) an essential question: "Is the couple relationship a resting place, a place that provides an experience where the 'objective object' each member has 'found,' is not at odds with the 'subjective object' that each of them has 'created?'" Does the relationship rest on the ground of this potentially generative, transfor-mational paradox?

## "Reality" and the experience (creative illusion) of feeling "real" in the couples

Midway into her paper, Friend takes up the complex question of the role of "reality" in couple work and theory:

> There is an implicit assumption throughout the literature that building healthy couple relating always involves a strengthened relationship including the capacity to bear disappointment, and what is generally referred to as disillusionment. We try to help couples see each other clearly and realistically. Couples are best equipped to weather the strains and changes in life if they can bear to mourn what is not possible, what has been lost, or what must be given up. All of this is in keeping with the task of encouraging and building capacities that are related to depression position functioning: the softening of omnipotence, the capacity to mourn, and the ability to feel genuine concern and empathy for a separate other.
>
> (this volume, p. 37)

Here, Friend is highlighting the importance of the "reality" dimension of couple life, found in Kleinian and neo-Kleinian thinking – the ways we must all come to terms with what isn't or can't be. I hear Friend implicitly suggesting that our work with couples would be impoverished if the best we could offer would be the ability to face one's losses together, to come to terms with the gap existing between the person we created and the one who is there, as we navigate the challenges of life together. Like Philips, Friend also notes that experiences of love cannot be accounted for in terms of depressive position functioning alone. Here we have a profound shift in emphasis in which the areas of illusion—and there are many in life – can get overly schematised. For Winnicott, the "reality" dimensions of the objective partner, as seen from the subjective experience of oneself, is of much less consequence, than the ways each member experiences themselves and the relationship as feeling "real." The "flesh" (Merleau-Ponty, 1968) of the experience of feeling real then returns us to the earlier discussion about the "ground" of being together. Referring to Winnicott's clock (Winnicott, 1986, p. 49), as referred to in Goldman (in press, quoted above, p. 6) he is "careful not to see clocks except just where he knows there already is one." Nonetheless, he created the clock. It became *his* clock. Here, he is punctuating the importance of what could be thought of as the primary narcissism (in the good sense) involved in primary creativity.

As Philips has pointed out, psychoanalysis "has an impoverished vocabulary for states of plenitude that are not considered pathological" (1993, p. 41). In this statement, Philips is staging a later debate about the significance of a "vitalizing presence" (Alvarez, 2012; Peltz, 2018, 2021; Schwartz-Cooney and Sopher, 2021) as a precursor to the ability to constitute "absence." Elsewhere I have written:

> These fleeting moments of lifeness animate our souls. They make life worth living. They hold the "truth" of our "own-most" fleeting and impossible-to-capture flashes of life … Infant researchers describe "action schemas," non-symbolic attentiveness, our operative vs. cultivated languages, and Ogden's ontological domain of being, which I think of as the beginning register of this vitalizing domain.
>
> (Peltz, 2021, p. 59)

In keeping with the spirit of transitional experiences, the experience of "realness" is always infused with the "to and fro of imaginative apperception and objective perception" (Goldman, in press). When the relationship comes to feel like a "real" resting place (even when it is stormy), then each member can feel themselves to be more than who they were before experiencing each other. I think of this as the "third" of the couple – when what grows between them is larger than the sum of each of them. Couples are able to "weave each other" (Winnicott, 1971, p. 3) into the "personal patterns" of who they are in a way that makes them more than who they were before they experienced each other (Ogden, 2019) – and that is a wonderful feeling.

## References

Alvarez, A. (2012). *The thinking heart: Three levels of psychoanalytic therapy with disturbed children.* New York: Routledge.

Bion, W. R. (1970). Attention and interpretation. In *Seven servants.* New York: Aronson.

Durbin, J. (2014). Despair and hope: On some varieties of countertransference and enactment in the psychoanalysis of ASD (Autistic spectrum disorder) children. *Journal of Child Psychotherapy,* 40(2), 187–200.

Eshel, O. (2013). Patient-analyst "withness": On analytic "presencing," passion and compassion in states of breakdown, despair and deadness. *Psychoanalytic Quarterly,* 82(4), 925–963.

Goldman, D. (in press). Winnicott's moon. In J. Aguayo (Ed.), *Winnicott in America.* Oxford University Press.

Goldner, V. (2017). Romantic bonds, binds, and ruptures: Couples on the brink. In S. Nathan & M. Schaefer (Eds.), *Couples on the couch: Psychoanalytic couple therapy and the Tavistock model* (pp. 154–179). London: Routledge.

Klein, M. (1930) The importance of symbol formation in the development of the ego. *International Journal of Psychoanalysis*, 11, 24–39.

Merleau-Ponty, M. (1968). *The visible and the invisible*. Evanston, IL: Northwestern University Press.

Morgan, M. (1995). The projective gridlock: A form of projective identification in couple relationships. In S. Ruszczynsky & J. Fisher (Eds.), *Intrusiveness and intimacy in the couple* (pp. 33–48). London: Karnac Books.

Morgan, M. (2005). On being able to be a couple: The importance of a "creative couple" in psychic life. In F. Grier (Ed.), *Oedipus and the couple* (pp. 9–30). London: Karnac.

Ogden, T. (2019). Ontological psychoanalysis or "what do you want to be when you grow up?" *Psychoanalytic Quarterly*, 88(4), 661–684.

Peltz, R. (2017). Discussion of "Romantic bonds, binds and ruptures: Couples on the brink". In S. Nathan & M. Schaefer (Eds.), *Couples on the couch: Psychoanalytic couple Therapy and the Tavistock Model* (pp. 180–192). London: Routledge.

Peltz, R. (2018). Discussion of "Vitalizing Enactment." *Psychoanalytic Dialogues*, 28, 361–370.

Peltz, R. (2021). Activating lifeness in the analytic encounter: The ground of being in psychoanalysis. In A. Schwartz-Cooney & R. Sopher (Eds.), *Vitalization in Psychoanalysis: Perspectives on being and becoming* (pp. 58–81). London: Routledge.

Person, E. S. (1988). *Dreams of love and fateful encounters*. New York: Penguin.

Phillips, A. (1993). *On kissing, tickling and being bored: Psychoanalytic essays on the unexamined life*. Cambridge, MA: Harvard University Press.

Phillips, A. (1994). *On flirtation*. Cambridge, MA: Harvard University Press.

Schwartz-Cooney, A. & Sopher, R. (Eds.). (2021). *Vitalization in psychoanalysis: perspectives on being and becoming*. New York: Routledge.

Winnicott, D. W. (1964). The baby as a growing concern. In D. W. Winnicott (Ed.), *The child, the family and the outside world*. Harmondsworth: Penguin Books.

Winnicott, D. W. (1971). Transitional objects and transitional phenomena. In *Playing and reality* (pp. 1–25). New York: Basic Books.

Winnicott, D. W. (1986). Living creatively. In C. Winnicott, R. Shepherd, & M. Davis (Eds.), *Home is where we start from: Essays by a psychoanalyst* (pp. 39–54). New York: W.W. Norton & Company.

Chapter 5

# Infidelity as manic defence

*Shelley Nathans*

## Introduction

The paths leading to infidelity are manifold and diverse; there is no singular cause, no simple, linear route. Rather, the complex set of psychological and interpersonal dynamics that influence and shape the events that lead to infidelity are unique to each relationship. The main focus of this chapter is on the problems that one or both of the partners in a couple may have with mourning past or impending loss, and the consequent infidelity that may result from a manic attempt to replace depression or psychic pain with excitement. In addition, I describe the role of unresolved pre-Oedipal and Oedipal issues and the ensuing triangulations that may develop, providing the psychic structures for infidelity. Using a Kleinian framework, I explore infidelity by examining the links between unresolved loss, unconscious triangulations, and the manic defences that may exist in couple relationships affected by affairs. In order to focus on this theoretical inquiry, I illustrate these ideas with an account of a couple who initiated psychotherapy in an attempt to cope with the crisis of infidelity.

## Problems with mourning loss and infidelity

Infidelity may reflect a range of psychological dilemmas across the developmental spectrum. Understanding any particular infidelity rests on exploring the specific nature of the unconscious phantasies and dynamic conflicts associated with that particular couple. This is where the work of the psychoanalytic couple psychotherapist lies – identifying the couple's unique set of dynamics that arise out of the intersection of each of the partners' internal object relations field,

DOI: 10.4324/9781003265023-5

their associated anxieties and defences, and the ways in which both the intrapsychic and interpersonal worlds mutually influence one another and create particular problems for that couple.

But even if there are myriad routes to infidelity – or to paraphrase the songwriter, Paul Simon – there must be fifty ways to cheat your lover – perhaps some unconscious paths might be more common than others. Over the years, I have noticed a recurrent theme in many of the couples coming for psychotherapy to cope with the crisis resulting from the revelation or discovery of an infidelity. Preceding the affair, there will be a significant un-metabolised loss, or series of losses, within the couple, and it is often the situation that one or both of the partners will not have made any link between the loss and the ensuing infidelity. Some obvious examples of these types of losses are: the loss of a job or large amount of money; the youngest child leaving home resulting in what is termed "the empty nest"; serious illness in the family; or the death of a parent or a child. Less blatant examples might revolve around developmental life changes that might provoke a sense of loss such as pregnancy, the birth of a child, retirement, or the physical and psychological declines of ageing.

In more disturbed couples, for example, those who tend to rely on action-oriented defensive strategies and have more comprehensive impediments to the capacity for mourning, an affair can easily offer an exciting distraction and manic defence against depression and pain. Infidelity can also occur in higher functioning couples who possess long histories of stability, satisfying sexual relations, and a capacity for mourning. When a severely traumatic loss, or series of losses, proves to be too much for the partners or the relationship to bear, these otherwise healthier relationships may not be sufficiently resilient to contain such immense pain, and this may result in one of the partners initiating an affair.

## The crisis of an affair

Typically, a maelstrom ensues when a couple finds themselves confronted with the mutual awareness of one of the partner's previously unknown infidelity. The couple finds themselves in crisis, attempting to manage many agonising feelings including shock, rage, betrayal, shame, humiliation, and guilt. The revelation of an infidelity tends to disrupt all previously held assumptions about the relationship and the sense of security about everyday life that had been shared. Often a dizzying sense of confusion descends upon them. What is true and what is a lie? Who can be trusted and who cannot be believed? And most importantly, what is real and what is not? (Elise, 2012).

This scenario will be all too familiar to any couple psychotherapist because it is a frequent presenting problem for those couples who are initiating treatment following the revelation or discovery of an affair. We are often called upon to help couples sort out this painful and traumatic confusion. There are many vital questions to be asked. How did this happen and why? What is the meaning of the affair and in what way is it experienced as a betrayal? Is this the first and only affair and are there other secrets or lies in the relationship? What aspects of the relationship have been irreparably broken and what might be restored? What is the role of forgiveness and remorse for a couple trying to recover from the revelation of an infidelity? Will it be possible for them to stay together, and develop renewed intimacy, or will the crisis inevitably lead to the end of the relationship? These questions were particularly relevant for me in the case of a couple whom I shall call Amy and Dave.

## Amy and Dave

It is Monday morning and I return the phone message of a new patient, Amy. Initially Amy is calm on the phone as we speak about the logistics of scheduling an appointment for her and her husband, Dave. Then, as her infant daughter starts crying in the background, Amy's voice breaks as she tells me the reason for coming to couple psychotherapy. She has just discovered that Dave has been having an affair. I can sense her fear, confusion, and the rising panic in her voice. She says she feels like there is no solid ground beneath her feet; it is difficult to breathe. She says she is in shock and she tells me that Dave is also in a state of turmoil. Neither of them has slept all night. Amy says she knows she has to remain focused on taking care of their children, a 3-year-old boy and the baby girl. It feels like the world has been unalterably changed and it is impossible to get her bearings. I shall return to this couple throughout the chapter to illustrate the theoretical concepts that I am discussing.

## Infidelity in context

It is necessary, although challenging, to understand infidelity without being moralistic. It would be too facile to dismiss all affairs
as purely pathological. Infidelities occur across the developmental
spectrum and can reflect a wide range of motives, both conscious
and unconscious. Conceptualised in this manner, it is possible to
think of some acts of infidelity as movements towards health –
for example, as developmental strivings to escape dead, loveless
relationships.

Moreover, the meaning of an extramarital affair differs widely from
one culture to the next. In certain countries and in some socio-eco-
nomic classes, an illicit affair is often not considered taboo or particularly threatening, while in others it is viewed as tantamount to the end
of the relationship. This variance in attitudes can also be observed in
certain subcultures, such as those engaged in mutually agreed upon
polyamorous relationships. Another example may be found in some
long-term, highly stable, gay male relationships that have an explicit
agreement that sexual encounters with other persons are permissible
and are not considered to be an infidelity.

It is still possible, however, for those with open relationships or
polyamorous couples to find themselves in a crisis of infidelity if one
of the partners breaks the explicit terms of the agreement. Infidelity
is a breach of an agreement about the nature of sexual boundaries
between the partners. Despite some couples' fantasies, expanding the
perimeter of the boundaries of a relationship does not necessarily
give immunity to these problems. For example, if a couple agrees
that they may have sex outside the relationship and one of the partners falls in love with someone else, this will be experienced as a
betrayal.

These types of open or polyamorous arrangements are the excep-
tion in modern romantic relationships, however, and most couples
view illicit sexual liaisons as extremely threatening because they represent a direct attack on the couple's link to one another. Since infidelities, by definition, are usually replete with dishonesty, betrayal, and
enormous pain, it would be unwise to ignore their inherent ubiquitous
aggressive and destructive aspects. Furthermore, from a psychoanalytic point of view, a primary task in a couple psychotherapy would be
to explore the link between unconscious anxieties and the defensive

attack on the couple that an affair might represent. I am proposing that in these cases, an exploration will frequently reveal a history of significant loss for the couple, and that infidelity has served as a powerful and exciting defence against mourning.

## Amy and Dave

Amy and Dave, the couple I described above, had experienced two major losses preceding Dave's affair, the most significant of which occurred when their oldest child was two. In the ninth month of Amy's second pregnancy, the baby died during delivery. This tragedy was made all the more difficult because it occurred without warning and the shock of the death of their baby was juxtaposed against the experience of innocence and hope they had felt during an otherwise normal, full-term pregnancy. There had been no time, no opportunity to prepare themselves for the impact of the trauma. Similarly, both Amy and Dave said they felt an absence of space and time to integrate and absorb the death of the baby. Approximately one year later, Amy was pregnant again and Dave's mother passed away. Despite the immense suffering and psychological dislocation that they each felt at the time, they found it difficult to talk to one another or grieve together. Amy felt pressure to return to the demands of her work and did not want to appear "too sad" because she believed that was best for their son. The distance between them grew and their bickering escalated into more frequent fights. Dave, acutely aware of their many financial obligations, retreated to his work life, where he found the comfort of a female co-worker and escaped the pain he felt at home.

## Theoretical conceptualisations in the psychoanalytic literature

Despite the widely recognised frequency with which infidelity occurs in many relationships, there is a dearth of writing about it in the psychoanalytical couple literature. There have, however, been a variety of psychoanalytic theoretical models for understanding infidelity, most of which centre on Oedipal problems that complicate the integration of both emotional and sexual intimacy in the couple relationship (Akhtar & Kramer, 1996; Elise, 2012; Josephs, 2006; Kernberg, 1995; Persons, 1988; Scharff & Scharff, 1991; Strean, 1980).

## The Oedipus complex and the contemporary family

Before describing the aspects of the Oedipus complex that are especially relevant to understanding infidelity, I want to briefly highlight an important theoretical limitation. In my view, there is a lag between psychoanalytic theory and the reality of present-day family life, where many families are not composed of two parents of the opposite sex. In this chapter, I am going to consider the Oedipus complex from a Kleinian view and attempt to use the model in a contemporary context, divorcing it from its historical heterosexist bias. Conceived in this more contemporary way, it is possible to apply Klein's ideas about the Oedipal Situation to non-traditional families with a single parent or two parents of the same sex. In these situations, the child must still come to terms with the anxieties and demands of the Oedipal Situation since frustration and loss of the primary parent will inevitably be a part of reality. There is no reason to assume that same-sex parental couples offer no less an opportunity for the psychological development associated with the depressive position and the achievement of triangular psychic space. Similarly, a child being raised with a single parent must come to recognise that they do not have exclusive possession of that parent due to the parent's relationship to other important persons or activities outside of the infant–parent dyad.

## The Kleinian view of the Oedipus complex

In contemporary Kleinian theory, both the ubiquity and necessity of negotiating the complexities of the Oedipal Situation are seen as central organising schema and this has important theoretical implications for understanding infidelity. Klein (1928) viewed the Oedipal Situation as beginning in early infancy, when the infant turns away from the mother in frustration and moves towards the father, creating the initial triangle constituted by the infant, mother, and father. For Klein, another aspect of Oedipal triangulation occurs through the child's confrontation with the awareness that the parents have a relationship. She argued that coming to terms with the recognition of the parental couple, the sexual link between them, and the reality of being excluded from this relationship, are all fundamental to the development of psychic functioning and the achievement of depressive position capacities. These depressive position capacities are associated with mature psychological and sexual functioning and have important implications for understanding infidelity.

If the child is able to accept the reality of the parental couple and tolerate being excluded from this dyad, a type of flexible triangulation can result (Britton, 1989) that allows for a form of linked separateness (Balfour, 2005). This creates the capacity to share psychic space, to maintain a sense of one's own separateness while, at the same time, being linked in relation to another without an overwhelming fear of being engulfed. From the depressive position, within this flexible triangular space, being excluded from the parental couple or its subsequent symbolic representations will not be experienced as catastrophic. The wish to attack and triumph over an internal parental couple will be diminished. Rivalry will be experienced as less destructive, will not be equated with death to the dyad, and will therefore be less anxiety producing. Consequently, there will be a more flexible capacity to integrate a symbolic or actual third because it will not be imbued with such threatening aspects. Thus, rather than engaging in denial, splitting, projection, and the enactment of unresolved Oedipal conflicts through the solution of infidelity, it will be more possible for a person to integrate sexual and emotional intimacy and introject a creative parental couple as an internal object (Frisch & Frisch-Desmarez, 2010; Morgan, 2005; Morgan & Freedman, 2009).

Traversing the complexities of the Oedipal Situation in a relatively less problematic way has other important implications for the capacity to form a creative couple relationship, maintain loyalty to it, and refraining from enacting unresolved Oedipal issues through infidelity. Since the Oedipal Situation requires a gradual relinquishment of the fantasy of exclusive possession of the desired parent, as well as acceptance of the reality of being excluded from the parental couple, this promotes an increased capacity to tolerate loss and results in a capacity for mourning.

Realistically, psychological development does not happen in a direct, unwavering, linear fashion. Rather, it is comprised of fits and starts: developmental progress and regression occur, along with the oscillation between paranoid schizoid and depressive position functioning. In fact, the psychic life of each person (and all couples) fluctuates between developmental and defensive functioning. However, when depressive position capacities are impaired, or have not been achieved, an individual will be more likely to rely on other defences to manage the anxieties and losses intrinsic to love relations: manic defences to replace pain with excitement, and projection and splitting to promote defensive triangulations in relationships.

### Splitting and triangulations in infidelity

A number of writers (Ehrhardt, 2006; Josephs, 2006; Kernberg, 1995; Persons, 1988; Strean, 1980) have emphasised a variety of ways that splitting and projection may underlie the triangulation inherent in infidelity, all of which are thought to spring from unresolved pre-Oedipal or Oedipal issues. Josephs (2006), following Freud, argues that unresolved Oedipal conflicts can give rise to defensive splitting because the child perceives parental intercourse as an act of infidelity. The child feels a sense of betrayal by the longed for, although unfaithful parent. This sense of betrayal promotes phantasies of revenge and a defensive organisation of splitting the desired parent into faithful and unfaithful parts. Hostility is projected onto the rivalrous parent and identification occurs with the desired one. The splitting promotes phantasies of escape from a bad object and union with an ideal one, leading to what Josephs (2006) terms "the impulse to infidelity."

The form of unconscious splitting in infidelity gets manifest in a triangulation involving the betrayed partner, the cheating partner, and the illicit lover. These triangulations, as I will subsequently describe, can serve a number of defensive purposes, including providing the organisation for the manic fantasy of escape from pain to an idealised sexual object. In my view, it is helpful to understand the unconscious structure of the triangulation of an affair, within the context of a manic defence against loss, as this is a complex formulation that explains both the especially compelling and painful aspects of infidelity. There are two types of basic triangulations that may be active unconsciously and underlie illicit liaisons: split-object triangles and rivalrous triangles (Person, 1988). As will be seen later in the case of Amy and Dave presented in this chapter, the two types of triangulations (split-object and rivalrous) may coexist but one type may predominate.

### Rivalrous triangulation

In a rivalrous split, there is a defensive reversal of the Oedipal triangulation. Instead of competing for the Oedipal object (for example, a child competing with one parent for the other parent's affection), the rivalrous triangulation of the adult affair reverses the Oedipal Situation. This puts the cheating spouse in a very powerful position. Rather than being the one who must compete and potentially lose the longed-for parent to a rival, they have now become the object of rivalry between the spouse and the lover. In addition, because the partner who commits the infidelity does not maintain exclusive loyalty to either his or her spouse or lover, the reverse triangulation creates an opportunity aggressively to enact unconscious revenge which may be obscured by intense guilt (Kernberg, 1995).

## Split-object triangulations

In contrast to the rivalrous triangulation, a split-object triangulation is based on the fantasy of a conflict free relationship with one ideal partner and one bad partner who represents an object who cannot provide what is longed for and needed. There are many possible forms of split-object triangulations representing a range of conflicts across the developmental spectrum. For example, a split-object triangulation might occur when the partner projects a pre-Oedipal mother, or a critical and punitive father, onto their spouse, from whom they must either escape or separate. In this type of scenario, the affair could represent, at one end of the developmental spectrum, a flight from the tyrannical grip of a restrictive and punitive object or an attempt to escape from a claustrophobic entrapment that threatens engulfment. The anxieties at the more disturbed end of the spectrum are thought to arise out of early failures in containment within the primary infant–parent relationship and these have an impact on the course of development through the Oedipal Situation, leaving their mark on psychic structures. Problems with sharing psychic space result and, consequently, there will be difficulties holding onto one's individual autonomy while being in a close relationship. The anxieties in this range include fears of annihilation, abandonment, fragmentation, and engulfment – those conceptualised in terms of autistic-contiguous anxieties or the agoraphobic/claustrophobic spectrum (Meltzer, 1992; Ogden, 1989; Rey, 1994), all of which will undoubtedly present serious impediments to the development of mature, stable romantic relationships (Balfour, 2005; Berg, 2012; de Marneffe, 2011).

In common parlance, we often refer to the initiation of a romantic relationship as "getting into" a relationship – a term that refers to the aspect of an intimate relationship that might be experienced as a type of symbolic container. On the other hand, if a relationship is experienced, quite concretely, more as a claustrophobic trap, rather than something that provides a sense of containment, then it will be very anxiety-provoking to "get into" a relationship. For a person struggling with these types of claustrophobic anxieties, an intimate relationship might induce a fear of "getting caught in" a relationship trap, rather than "getting into" an intimate relationship. These same anxieties can serve as a powerful propellant to get out of the trap, to flee the threat of engulfment. Similarly, having an illicit affair – a relationship "on the side" – can serve as a defensive solution that enables an individual to remain in an otherwise "committed" relationship. Infidelity often serves as a readily available and convenient way out of such a claustrophobic relationship dilemma.

Moving away from the more disturbed end of the developmental spectrum, a split-object triangulation could arise as a defensive attempt to manage a different level of anxiety. For example, conflict over incestuous longings and unconscious guilt might prevent one or both of the partners from the psychic freedom to form their own parental couple (Morgan, 2005) or to have sexual enjoyment in their relationship. One solution to this conflict is to de-sexualise the spouse through projection, for example when one partner transforms his or her spouse into an asexual sibling or parental object. This serves to diminish erotic desire and leads the partner to seek freedom outside the marriage in a sexual liaison that forms a triangulation with one de-sexualised spouse and a forbidden sexual lover (Strean, 1980).

## Amy and Dave

An example of the projections that lay the seeds for a split-object triangulation can be found in the case of the couple described in this chapter, Amy and Dave. Dave consciously identified himself as a "teenage man." Many of the marital tensions between them, even predating the deaths of their baby and his mother, involved conflicts over his wishes to be liberated from the responsibilities of their life together. He felt oppressed by having to support the family financially and resented Amy's requests for help when he was at home. He wanted to go snowboarding during the winter, play Frisbee with friends, or go out with the guys.

Amy had grown up with the feeling that she was never understood by her parents and often felt very lonely as a child. She had been adopted at birth and reported feeling like she was a stranger in her own home, where there was a polite, distant formality. Her parents employed a full-time nanny and she attended boarding schools beginning at age fourteen. She said that she had always been accustomed to taking care of herself emotionally. Determined to not be like her own parents, she devoted herself to taking care of her children. Feeling alone and tethered to two small children, she grew increasingly angry and resentful while Dave was out "having fun." This experience recreated the isolated feeling she had as a child and she increasingly withdrew from Dave, both sexually and emotionally.

Dave felt that Amy spent all of her time and energy with the children and had little left over for him. One the one hand, he felt jealous of their children who seemed to get all the attention at his expense, and on the other hand, he was furious that she acted like "the boss of the house" and denied him active participation regarding important decisions, which kept him in a childlike position. This situation painfully repeated the experiences of his childhood when his mother had been very ill and unavailable during the first three years of his life. Like Amy, Dave had felt deprived of emotional contact from a very early age and he felt that he had to learn to take care of himself. He grew up in a strict, Catholic family and had attended parochial schools with Nuns whom he experienced as draconian and authoritarian. Not surprisingly, Dave experienced Amy as a rigid, controlling parental figure to whom he had to submit. He felt she criticised him when he didn't comply with her rules and he experienced her withdrawal as a form of punishment. He felt trapped by Amy, by his adult responsibilities and by his marriage.

Before the traumatic loss of their baby and the death of Dave's mother, the problematic dynamics of their relationship existed between them in a corrosive, yet stable way. Their difficulties were ensconced in the aspects of the relationship that they regarded as valuable. Following these losses, these problems became the foreground of their relationship, eclipsing and destroying any good feelings between them.

## Mourning

A thorough discussion of the psychoanalytic theory of mourning is beyond the scope of this chapter, but it is important to highlight some aspects of the theory that are relevant to understanding how difficulties with mourning may be associated with the impulse to infidelity.

In Freud's earliest contributions to this topic, detailed in *Mourning and Melancholia* (1917e, [1915]), he juxtaposed two possible psychological responses to loss that follow an initial period of grief: normal mourning and melancholia. Freud outlined a theory of the internal process of identifications that occur in the mind of the mourner that allow him or her, over time, to gradually overcome their loss. In contrast, Freud argued that melancholia, what we might today term severe depression or pathological mourning, occurs instead of a normal mourning process. Therefore, for a person with difficulties accepting the reality of loss, melancholia takes over when mourning is not possible. When problems with mourning occur within the couple, in one or both of the partners, it will be more difficult for them to share the reality of the loss, turn to one another for support, and rely on the relationship as a resource for containment of the painful feelings. Conceptualised in these terms, we might think of a melancholic couple replacing a mourning couple.

In the Kleinian model, negotiation of the Oedipal Situation, and the related development of the depressive position, creates a capacity for mourning (Klein, 1940). This capacity rests primarily and fundamentally on the individual's relation to reality – on the ability to recognise and accept loss, as opposed to defensively deny it. For both Freud and Klein, difficulties with coming to terms with the reality of loss result in the mobilisation of defensive processes. Freud emphasised the splitting of the ego that allows a person to both know and not know that they have suffered a loss (Quinodoz, 2007; Steiner, 2005). Kernberg (2010) has emphasised that normal mourning involves an internal object relationship with the lost object that promotes identification and superego development, both of which are necessary for maintaining stable and faithful sexual relationships. It is easy to see how both superego deficits, as well as, the splitting of the ego may operate in many infidelities, where it is possible for the unfaithful partner to both know and not know what they are doing. They may experience intense erotic desire and excitement when they are with their lover, all the while keeping the anxiety and pain they may otherwise feel about cheating or getting caught out of awareness.

## Manic defence

One of the significant contributions of Kleinian theory is the elaboration of the concept of the manic defence (Klein, 1935, 1940, 1945).

For Freud, mania is an escape from melancholia. For Klein, mania involves both a massive denial of reality and an attempt to escape from the frightening awareness of our vulnerability and dependency on others, resulting in a desperate drive to find freedom (Klein, 1935).

Klein theorised the manic defence as a mechanism of overactivity that serves to manage the anxieties associated with the depressive position: the experience of loss, vulnerability, dependency, limitation, and the awareness of time and mortality. Manic defences are based on a detachment from psychic reality and rely on omnipotence, denial, and idealisation. The omnipotence replaces concern for others with control; the denial obscures the awareness of dependency on others, and the idealisation splits psychic experience to foster the fantasy of an all-good, perfect experience without pain. Manic defences also obscure and obliterate the superego and provide a defence against guilt and the recognition of one's own destructive capacities (Bronstein, 2010).

Acts of infidelity rely profoundly on the manic defence because this dynamic provides both an idealised object in the form of an illicit lover and the illusion of escape from pain. Simultaneously, the manic defence permits one to deny an awareness of dependency on a partner to whom one is faithfully committed, as well as, the pain and destructive potential of the infidelity. Unresolved pre-Oedipal and Oedipal issues result in triangulations and provide the psychic structures underlying acts of infidelity, and manic defences supply the intoxicating fuel that propels them.

## Amy and Dave

After the baby died, Amy threw herself into her work and the caretaking of their son, a relationship in which she found comfort. She said that she was very sad about the loss of the baby but wanted to get pregnant again as soon as possible. This idea was encouraged and supported by both of the couple's extended families and it was justified in their minds with the rationale that it would be better for their family to "move on." During this time, Amy experienced Dave as even more physically active and unavailable. He was often away from home, travelling for work or involved with sports. When he was at home, he was surly and he began to drink more. She said that she remembered thinking that he was absent even when he was present.

Dave also experienced Amy as unavailable. From his point of view, she was always preoccupied with work or taking care of their son. He reported trying to reach out to Amy, wanting to be closer to her and their son and more involved with parenting and decisions regarding the family. He said he longed for more of a shared life together as a couple and as a family, but he felt that Amy "pushed him away" and that she was always critical of him and angry. Their sexual contact during this time felt perfunctory and pragmatic as it was organised around the attempt to get pregnant again. He said he felt like the baby monkey with the wire mother in the famous Harlow experiment. He had tried to seek comfort from Amy but found her to be cold and unresponsive to his needs.

Dave's experience of Amy as a cold and unresponsive maternal object – a wire mother – formed one side of a split-object triangulation and in distinction to his experience of the woman with whom he had the affair, a much younger, single woman who had no obligations and was always at the ready to meet him at a moment's notice. The excitement of the sexual contact with the lover stood in stark contrast to the token and mechanistic sex he experienced at home, which he felt was commanded by Amy according to her ovulation cycles. In Dave's mind, Amy became a cold, unavailable maternal object to him. At the same time, he felt he was in competition for her affection with their son, who seemed to get everything he wanted from Amy. This psychic arrangement resulted in two triangulations in Dave's mind: one formed by Dave's exclusion from the dyadic relationship between Amy and their son and the other formed by the triangle of Amy, Dave, and the lover, a defensive solution that provided revenge, comfort for his unbearable pain, and a manic retreat for Dave.

On Amy's part, there also formed a defensive triangulation and a manic defence. She sought retreat and consolation in the dyadic relationship with her son, reversing the roles such that she experienced the boy as giving comfort to her. From within this split-object triangulation, it was not possible for her to be close to both Dave and their son. The son was idealised and Dave vilified – he was the bad child, the non-compliant, teenage man who left her on her own to figure out everything by herself, a figure with whom she was familiar from her childhood.

Amy and Dave colluded in their attempts to avoid the pain of the loss of the baby with the manic defence of achieving an immediate replacement pregnancy. Due to each of their deficits in the capacity for mourning, they were not able to turn to one another or rely on their couple relationship in their grief. It was striking that they both recalled wanting to turn to the other for solace but found an unavailable partner.

Along with the painful loss of the baby, the shared manic defences also served to ward off anxiety about another pregnancy. Dave said that he had felt terrified that they might lose another baby when Amy got pregnant again, but he didn't feel they had ever been able to talk about this fear together. Amy said she hadn't been too worried since the first pregnancy had been successful, they had a healthy boy, and the doctors had assured them that the odds of such a tragedy recurring were very small. She experienced Dave's anxiety as oppositional and unnecessarily negative; she said she didn't see the point in focusing on what might go wrong.

The manic defensive organisation of this couple prevented them from awareness of their own anxieties and pain, as well as the pain and anxiety in one another. It wasn't possible for Dave to think of Amy as a grieving mother, as someone who had been through a terrible trauma and shared his pain, or to see the side of her that was trying to be a good mother, as a mother resisting the pull of depression that might result in the neglect of their son. From the position of the split, he projected onto her a cold, critical, unavailable and mechanistic "wire" mother. Because he felt so needy, like the monkey in the experiment, he could not acknowledge Amy's needs. Similarly, Amy could not see Dave's pain, loneliness, or desperation. She only experienced him as someone who was wilfully misunderstanding and neglecting her. She projected her own needs to be taken care of into him and experienced him as a selfish, non-compliant, teenage man. She could not see the side of Dave that was striving to be a responsible husband and concerned father.

The combination of these projective processes, their split-object triangulations, the limitations in their capacities for mourning, and their reliance on manic defences left them extremely psychologically vulnerable when faced with the task of absorbing traumatic loss. Distance and anger replaced mutual vulnerability and dependency needs. Triangulations, based on rigid projections and splits, provided temporary, idealised retreat. Pressured activity replaced pain, emptiness, fear, and the awareness of loss.

## Conclusion

Loss is a ubiquitous fact of life and it is certain that every couple will have to come to terms with numerous losses throughout their lives together. When each partner has a capacity for mourning, they will be more likely to face loss in a shared way and experience their relationship as a source of containment. However, when there are deficits in the capacity for mourning in one or both of the partners, difficulties in facing their losses individually, and together, will more likely lead to defensive enactments that serve to deny loss, leading either to severe depression (melancholia) or to manic defences. In these circumstances, infidelity may serve as a possible vehicle for the manic attempt to deny both dependency and loss, and to replace pain with excitement. In some couples, the betrayed spouse's response to the revelation of the affair may also have manic defensive aspects. Unrelenting, indignant rage may sometimes serve as a manic correlate that defends against vulnerability and the awareness of loss, perpetuating the couple's dilemma.

Couple psychotherapy can offer such a couple an alternative – an opportunity to understand the complex processes that have engendered their crisis, as well as the possibility either to work through their difficulties or make the decision to separate. The couple presented in this chapter, Amy and Dave, worked for three years in weekly couple psychotherapy. The initial phase of the therapy focused on the anxiety and pain ensuing from the shock of the revelation of the affair. As the therapy progressed, they were increasingly able to speak together about the other painful loss in their lives – the death of their baby. Over time, they each began to understand their own contributions to the problems in their relationship and how their shared difficulties facing loss helped to create the conditions for the affair. They worked hard to change the dynamics in their relationship and, because they were motivated by a desire to keep the family intact for their children, they decided to stay together.

Although it may not be possible for all couples, many will be able to use couple psychotherapy to help them manage the crisis of the affair and develop an understanding of the unconscious dynamics that may have contributed to the problems in their relationship that preceded and lead to the infidelity. Under such circumstances, it may be more possible for the couple to gradually develop and relate with more depressive position capacities: acceptance of the reality of boundaries and limitations, greater tolerance for disappointments in themselves and their partner, increased empathic concern, awareness of individual responsibility, and remorse about the infidelity. With the containment offered in couple psychotherapy, it may be more possible for each of the partners to develop a greater capacity for mourning and together face the painful realities inherent in both past and future losses. Without such help, in the absence of containment, manic defences offer their seductions for the taking.

## References

Akhtar, S. & Kramer, S. (Eds.) (1996). *Intimacy and infidelity*. Northvale, NJ and London: Jason Aronson.

Balfour, A. (2005). The couple, their marriage, and Oedipus: or, problems come in twos and threes. In: F. Grier (Ed.), *Oedipus and the couple* (pp. 49–72). London: Karnac Books.

Berg, J. (2012). "A bad moment with the light." No-sex couples: the role of autistic-contiguous anxieties. *Couple and Family Psychoanalysis*, 2: 33–48.

Britton, R. (1989). The missing link: parental sexuality in the Oedipus complex. In: J. Steiner (Ed.), *The Oedipus Complex today: Clinical implications* (pp. 83–101). London: Karnac Books.

Bronstein, C. (2010). Two modalities of manic defences: their function in adolescent breakdown. *The International Journal of Psychoanalysis*, 91: 583–600.

de Marneffe, D. (2011). Marriage and lovesick yearning: internal boundaries, external limits. Unpublished manuscript.

Ehrhardt, W. (2006). Couples in narcissistic collusion: sexual fantasy and acting out. In: J. S. Scharff & D. E. Scharff (Eds.), *New paradigms for treating relationships* (pp. 345–359). Lanham, MD: Jason Aronson.

Elise, D. (2012). The danger in deception: Oedipal betrayal and the assault on truth. *Journal of the American Psychoanalytic Association*, 60(4), 679–705.

Freud, S. (1917e [1915]). *Mourning and Melancholia*, S. E. 14. 237–257.

Frisch, S. & Frisch-Desmarez, C. (2010). Some thoughts on the concept of the internal parental couple. *The International Journal of Psychoanalysis*, 91: 325–342.

Josephs, L. (2006). The impulse to infidelity and oedipal splitting. *The International Journal of Psychoanalysis*, 87: 423–437.

Kernberg, O. (1995). *Love relations: Normality and pathology*. New Haven, CT: Yale University Press.

Kernberg, O. (2010). Some observations on the process of mourning. *The International Journal of Psychoanalysis*, 91: 601–619.

Klein, M. (1928). Early stages of the oedipus conflict. *International Journal of Psycho-Analysis*, 9: 167–180 [Reprinted in: *Love, Guilt and Reparation & Other Works*, London: Hogarth Press, 1975].

Klein, M. (1935). A contribution to the psychogenesis of manic-depressive states. *International Journal of Psycho-Analysis*, 16: 145–174 [Reprinted in: *Love, Guilt and Reparation & Other Works*, London: Hogarth Press, 1975].

Klein, M. (1940). Mourning and its relation to manic-depressive states. *International Journal of Psycho-Analysis*, 21: 125–153 [Reprinted in: *Love, Guilt and Reparation & Other Works*, London: Hogarth Press, 1975].

Klein, M. (1945). The Oedipus Complex in the light of early anxieties. *International Journal of Psycho-Analysis*, 26: 11–33 [Reprinted in: *Love, Guilt and Reparation & Other Works*, London: Hogarth Press, 1975].

Meltzer, D. (1992). *The claustrum: An investigation of claustrophobic phenomena.* Perthshire: Clunie Press.

Morgan, M. (2005). On being able to be a couple: the importance of a "creative couple" in psychic life. In: F. Grier (Ed.), *Oedipus and the couple* (pp. 9–30). London: Karnac Books.

Morgan, M. & Freedman, J. (2009). From fear of intimacy to perversion. In: C. Clulow (Ed.), *Sex, attachment and couple psychotherapy* (pp. 185–198). London: Karnac Books.

Ogden, T. (1989). *The primitive edge of experience.* Northvale, NJ: Jason Aronson.

Person, E. (1988). *Dreams of love and fateful encounters: The power of romantic passion.* New York: W.W. Norton. [Reprinted Arlington, VA: American Psychiatric Publishing, 2007].

Quinodoz, J. M. (2007). Teaching Freud's "Mourning and Melancholia." In: L. Fiorinia, T. Bokanowski, & S. Lewkowicz (Eds.), *On Freud's 'Mourning and melancholia'* (pp. 179–192). London: Karnac Books.

Rey, H. (1994). *Universals of psychoanalysis in the treatment of psychotic and borderline states.* London: Free Association Books.

Scharff, J. S. & Scharff, D. E. (1991). *Object relations couple therapy.* Northvale, NJ: Jason Aronson.

Steiner, J. (2005). The conflict between mourning and melancholia. *Psychoanalytic Quarterly*, 74: 83–104.

Strean, H. (1980). *The extramarital affair.* Northvale, NJ: Jason Aronson.

# Chapter 6

# Discussion of "Infidelity as manic defence"

*Mary Morgan*

Nathans' chapter, "Infidelity as manic defence," originally published in 2012, is an important study in the couple psychoanalytic literature. The link she makes, borne out of her clinical experience, between unmetabolised loss, manic defences, and infidelity is convincing and clinically useful.

Infidelity is a challenging presentation in couple analysis because the couple are often very split into the victim and transgressor. Pressures may be put on the therapist to side with one partner against the other, to interrogate the partner who has had the affair, or to make moral judgements. The therapist has the difficult task of trying to understand the infidelity as occurring in the context of the relationship, while at the same time not ignoring and being attuned to the pain inflicted by the event of the infidelity on one partner by the other. Often there is the sense of the whole basis of the relationship crumbling, along with anxieties about what is real, and a breakdown in trust, which is sometimes irretrievable.

The therapist can feel recruited into the paranoid and manic dynamic that the couple feel thrown into. She can feel under pressure to join the couple in making rapid decisions about the future of the relationship. There is often a pressure for all the details of the infidelity to be revealed that can turn the therapy into some kind of interrogation. It can be difficult to steer a way through this and help the couple towards a state of mind in which they can look at what has happened to them as a couple, including links to unprocessed loss. The couple cannot quickly get themselves into this more reflective place. Usually, some time has to be spent on the concrete experience of the infidelity and acknowledgement of the pain caused before this work can take place. But with the configuration of the couple therapy,

DOI: 10.4324/9781003265023-6

the couple does have a special opportunity, in that now there is a different kind of third in the room – a person who, instead of siding with one of them can make room for the experience of each of them and focus on the crisis in their relationship, a third person who can bring a couple state of mind (Morgan, 2001, 2019). The link that Nathans makes between infidelity and an unmourned loss embedded in the fabric of the couple's relationship, can help a couple gradually move from a state of blame and accusation, denial, and defensiveness, to one in which they can begin to mourn and work through painful loss together, eventually, for some, giving an enlarged meaning to the infidelity.

Underpinning her thinking about infidelity as a manic defence, Nathans draws attention to the Oedipal Situation. First, she points out that the dynamics of the Oedipal triangular situation "provides the psychic structures underlying acts of infidelity and manic defences supply the intoxicating fuel that propels them" (Nathans, this volume, p. 69). "Rivalrous" and "split object triangulations," familiar and unresolved from the Oedipal Situation are brought to life and enacted once again, but this time triumphantly reversed. Further, she highlights the post-Kleinian view that working through the Oedipal Situation goes hand in hand with working through the depressive position. This is a continual process, as Britton describes,

> The depressive position and the Oedipus situation are never finished but have to be reworked in each new life situation, at each stage of development and with each major addition to experience of knowledge.
>
> (1992, p. 38)

Thus, managing loss is both aided by, and further reworks, the depressive position. Temperley (2001) reminds us that Klein described the work of mourning required with every major loss and disappointment as, "rebuilding with anguish the inner world." Temperley notes,

> This is particularly difficult where the depressive position has been precariously established in the first place and leaves the personality in danger of regression to the defences of the paranoid schizoid or to undue mobilization of a defence more specific to the depressive position, mania.
>
> (2001, p. 50)

One of the discoveries that couple analysts have made is that the adult couple relationship can be a powerful fulcrum for reworking earlier unmetabolised experience – internal object relationships, internal conflicts, or unrepresented primitive experience which resurface in different forms later in life. An area that gets psychic traction in an intimate adult couple relationship is the potential to re-experience the phantasy of the ideal object, the feeling of having found the "one," manifested at the beginning in the falling in love state of mind. Thus, while choosing to be part of a couple and relinquishing the pleasures and freedoms of single life or the exclusive ties to family of origin can, for many, feel to be an important psychological achievement, paradoxically, the falling in love state also contains elements of regression.

Following Nathans links to the Oedipal Situation, an aspect I will develop further is the experience of loss in the Oedipal Situation *itself*, the painful loss of the idealised primary object and the feeling of betrayal that comes with the awareness that there was another relationship that existed all along with the primary object's adult partner. This loss and disillusionment come early in development and is hard to metabolise at the time, thus it is probably only ever partially worked through. The falling in love state of mind and the re-finding of, and ultimate loss of, the ideal object, provides the conditions within which this earlier loss can be further worked through from a position of greater ego strength and maturity. However, the feelings re-evoked add intensity to current experiences and the current experience rekindles the earlier raw loss.

Elise describes this après coup aspect in relation to the Oedipal experience,

> I see in Oedipal betrayal a subjective experience of temporality where meaning travels backward and suffuses one's object-relational past, creating a new history that is now personally registered (though not "remembered") as immensely painful.
>
> (Elise, 2012, p. 690)

The earlier, always to some extent, unresolved relationship to the idealised object exerts a powerful force in the unconscious and provides the "fuel" (to use Nathans' word) to make the step into a new adult intimacy with the ideal other. The disillusionment of the ideal other and the idealised relationship provides further fuel to the ongoing work of the depressive position.

The partners must start to come to terms with who the other is and who they are as a couple, a different and more reality-based version to the idealised one. The psychic development that takes place in the relationship further works through the loss of the idealised pre-Oedipal object and the idealised primary relationship. Facing this loss, and all the feelings attached to it, allows new and unanticipated aspects of the other to be engaged with, and allows the relationship to develop and deepen.

In focusing on this inevitable form of loss in a couple relationship, I am not simply adding to the more tangible range of losses that a couple may experience – both in the couple life cycle and those losses that are unexpected and traumatic – but expanding the links that Nathans makes to the early Oedipal Situation. I suggest that unresolved early Oedipal loss, re-cathected in the adult intimate relationship, may intensify current losses, especially those which repeat the Oedipal configuration, such as those inherent to infidelity

## Loss and disillusionment in a couple relationship

If the loss of the ideal primary object can be managed, a more realistic perception of that object as containing good and bad aspects becomes possible. In an intimate adult couple there is the potential for further psychic development: a developing awareness of who the other is; who one is oneself, as seen reflected back by the other; and what the relationship can and cannot be. Cohen, in a recent article in the Guardian, cites Dorothea Brookes lament in George Eliot's *Middlemarch*, suggesting that there is something quite difficult in coming face to face with the other as they are.

> Marriage is so unlike anything else. There is something even awful in the nearness it brings.
>
> (2021, p. 22)

The nearness of the other, something that many couples have experienced during the recent pandemic, has for some been extremely challenging. The blind spots we have about the other – our capacity to "turn a blind eye" – is tested as the other comes into closer focus. For some, this has led to greater intimacy, but for others it has had a destabilising effect on their relationship as there is no escape from those avoided aspects of the other. As well as that, couples are faced over time, with or without the proximity that lockdowns create, with the otherness of the other.

Cohen suggests the essential paradox of intimacy is that,

> in intensifying our closeness to another, we not only make them more familiar to us; we come alive to their strangeness and irreducible difference.
>
> (2021, p. 23)

We were confronted with the otherness of the other early on when the ideal primary object was revealed to have another life, outside our orbit, a life going on all the time of which we had been unaware. Nevertheless, many couple analysts have observed that this reality can remain an intractable problem in relationships. For example, Puget believed that,

> To work with the complexity of links as it happens with family and couple psychoanalysis has to do with the difficulty to accept the unavoidable otherness and alienness of each one.
>
> (2019, p. 25)

The process of disillusionment is lived out in the everyday life of the couple. The other is revealed as not all we imagined they were, or who we thought we needed them to be. They can meet some of our needs but are unable or chose not to meet others. Their "nearness" brings the discovery that they are a challenging mixture of things. There is the loss of the phantasy about the relationship. As Vorchheimer argues,

> People not only fall in love with partners, but with the narcissistic representation of their togetherness, their love. Therefore, couples do not need an actual loss to occur in order to have an experience of perceived loss in relation to their link. Insofar as illusions can only maintain a temporary hold, the occurrence of certain everyday events can become a manifestation of the loss of their shared inaugural illusion.
>
> (2015, p. 132)

The loss that comes with disillusionment is also the point that new developments can take place in a couple relationship. The otherness of the other can lead to new discoveries for the self and creative possibilities in the relationship. Alternatively, the ideal object might be precariously held onto, but life events await to threaten its dissolution. One of the events that is particularly powerful in a couple relationship is pregnancy. The arrival of a baby, in which phantasy of the ideal object is challenged can cause a resurgence of Oedipal dynamics.

## Amy and Dave

Nathans brings a rich understanding to the unconscious dynamics between Dave and Amy, showing the ways in which, through their projective system, they live out in their relationship painful aspects of their shared internal worlds.

Dave identified himself as the "teenage man," feeling oppressed by supporting the family financially and experiencing Amy as demanding and controlling when at home. His mother had been ill and unavailable when he was young, and his family and school life were strict and draconian. He felt Amy started to embody these restrictive and cold earlier object relationships.

Amy had felt isolated as a child and being determined not to repeat this with her own children, she devoted herself to them, and by doing so, met some of her own emotional needs. She also grew angry and resentful of Dave's "freedom" and withdrew from Dave emotionally and sexually. His unavailability also repeated her earlier experience. One imagines the understanding that Nathans brings to these unconscious couple dynamics would be part of the enlarged perspective regarding the infidelity that she brought to bear in the process of the couple therapy.

Rather than further exploring the clinical material along these lines, I will highlight aspects of the given material that might point to the underlying early Oedipal loss I have been discussing. I am not suggesting that these links should be make directly to the couple. By understanding and working with the intensity of feelings associated with the current losses in the here and now, there will be, through the après coup, a further working through of the earlier loss.

For the couple therapist, understanding loss in a couple relationship as it relates to the profound, and only partially worked through, earlier loss of the ideal object and Oedipal betrayal, may serve to remind us of the intensity of the affect we encounter over particular kinds of loss. It helps us to understand why infidelity in particular has such a deep unconscious resonance and why it can be hard to work through and recover from. As Amy conveyed in the initial phone call,

> It feels like the world has been unalterably changed and it is impossible to get her bearings.
>
> (Nathans, this volume, p. 59)

The Oedipal dynamics of loss, exclusion, and betrayal are felt painfully by Amy in the affair, but this was present for both of them and problematic in their relationship before this occurred. Amy already felt excluded by Dave's life outside the home with work and friends, Dave felt excluded by Amy's relationship with the children. At the point whereby the couple might have grieved together the loss of their second child and deepened their relationship, they had already lost the other as a reliable, available presence. Disillusionment crashed in on this relationship as Amy became the Harlow's monkey wire mother for Dave, and Dave became the abandoning parent for Amy.

The longing for an ideal object can be more urgent when this was not provided earlier on, or if the Oedipal disillusionment comes at a point when there had not been a sufficient internalisation of a good object, one that will help in the working through of the depressive position.

Nathans observed that for Dave and Amy,

> Triangulations, based on rigid projections and splits, provided temporary, idealized retreat.
>
> (this volume, p. 71)

Each turned to another "ideal" object, Dave to the "much younger, single woman who had no obligations and was always ready to meet him at a moment's notice" (this volume p. 70) and Amy sought retreat and consolation in the dyadic idealised relationship with her first-born son.

Couple psychoanalytic theory postulates that within the conscious choice of partner there are significant unconscious elements in a couple's attraction to one another. We can imagine that this couple recognised in each other a core experience of a lack of emotional contact, aloneness, and isolation. They may have unconsciously sought to create a different kind of relationship together in which they would be emotionally available for each other, just as Amy sought to be for their children. The recognition, at a deep level, of difficult shared earlier experience may have provided them with a developmental possibility to work this through instead of repeating it in their own relationship. One wonders if this might have been possible had they not been confronted with traumatic loss that exacerbated their vulnerabilities? We don't know, but Nathans' feeling is that this couple did not have the psychic structure of sufficient depressive position capacity to work through loss without help. For example, she notes that instead,

> Amy and Dave colluded in their attempts to avoid the pain of the loss of the baby with the manic defence of achieving an immediate replacement pregnancy.
>
> (Nathans, this volume, p. 70)

The loss of a baby is a loss that hits a couple relationship at its core. As well as the profound loss of the baby itself, it can rock the couple's sense of themselves as being a creative couple (Morgan, 2005). In some couples, it can evoke paranoid feelings of having done something wrong and feeling punished, or a feeling that there is something wrong with the relationship. For this couple, a traumatic loss came at a time when they were already struggling to work through the ordinary developmental losses of the ideal object and relationship.

For some couples, particularly if they are spared traumatic loss, the unresolved Oedipal Situation is further worked through and strengthened in different ways, for example, through managing ordinary disappointment, inclusion, and exclusion, acceptance of the other's and one's own good and bad parts, and in a deepening loving bond towards a more or less "real" other.

## Conclusion

For any couple, there is a delicate balance between how much has been worked through early in each partner's life and what internal psychic structures are in place; how far the couple have progressed in their psychic development together; and what life events they are faced with, especially if they are traumatic in nature.

I agree with Nathans that many examples of infidelity are triggered by an experience of loss, and what could be described as a manic flight away from the loss. The loss that seems central is the loss of the ideal object and the manic flight is an attempt to rediscover the lost ideal object. Some individuals cannot give up the search for the ideal object and a phantasised ideal relationship, resulting in many affairs or many relationships. Some partners cannot recover from the experience of infidelity. They are left with a precarious sense of what is real and the breakdown of trust, feelings heightened by earlier Oedipal experience, and they choose to end the relationship. For others, the shock of the infidelity, the loss, the betrayal, and pain, can provide an opportunity to work, and re-work, through the loss of the ideal object and idealised relationship, instead of turning to manic solutions.

# References

Britton, R. (1992) Chapter 3: The Oedipus situation and the depressive position. In: R. Anderson (Ed.), *Clinical lectures in Klein and Bion* (pp. 34–45). London and New York: Tavistock/Routledge.

Cohen, J. (2021) *The Guardian Review*, Sunday March 2021, Issue No.165.

Elise, D. (2012). The danger in deception: Oedipal betrayal and the assault on truth. *Journal of the American Psychoanalytic Association*, 60(4), 679–705.

Morgan, M. (2001). First contacts: The therapist's "couple state of mind" as a factor in the containment of couples seen for initial consultations. In: F. Grier (Ed.), *Brief encounters with couples* (pp. 17–32). London: Karnac.

Morgan, M. (2005) On being able to be couple: The *importance* of a "creative couple" in psychic life. In: F. Grier (Ed.), *Oedipus and the couple* (pp. 9–30). London: Karnac Books.

Morgan, M. (2019) *A couple state of mind: Psychoanalysis of couples and the Tavistock Relationships Model*. London and New York: Routledge.

Nathans, S. (2012) Infidelity as manic defence. *Couple and Family Psychoanalysis*, 2(2) Autumn, 165–180. London: Karnac.

Puget, J. (2019) Chapter 1: Approaches to interpretation. In: T. Keogh and E. Palacios (Eds.), *Interpretation in couple and family psychoanalysis: Cross- cultural perspectives* (p. 25). London and New York: Routledge.

Temperley, J. (2001) Chapter 4: The depressive position. In: C. Bronstein (Ed.), *Kleinian theory: A contemporary perspective* (pp. 47–62). London and Philadelphia: Whurr Publishers.

Vorchheimer, M. (2015). Understanding the loss of understanding. *Paper presented at the IPA Congress*, Boston.

# Chapter 7

# Viewing the absence of sex from couple relationships through the "core complex" lens

*Amita Sehgal*

## Introduction

The sexual relationship is a defining feature of most intimate couple partnerships. Consequently, when sexual problems arise, couples become aware that something is amiss in the relationship that can no longer be ignored (Glasser, 1979). When couples experiencing problems in their sexual relationship seek treatment by approaching an agency that specialises in providing couple therapy, it is likely that the therapists will view the sexual dysfunction as evidence of emotional disturbance in the relationship as a whole.

This chapter describes how psychoanalytic psychotherapy has been used in the treatment of two clinical cases in which the absence of sex was a shared feature. In both cases, the couples sought therapeutic help with improving the quality of their relationship, and not psychosexual treatment. In working with sexual problems therapists can differ in their responses. For instance, clinicians focusing on physiology and performance may focus on medical aspects of an individual's experience to treat the functional aspects of sexual behaviour (a tendency encouraged by the categorisation of sexual dysfunction in the American Psychiatric Association's *Diagnostic and Statistical Manuals*). Therapeutic interventions may then be body-focused and directed at biochemical factors affecting sexual responses. More likely in the psychotherapy field are psychosexual approaches that take account of psychological and relationship factors too (see, e.g., Green & Seymour, 2009), including desensitising techniques for managing sexual anxiety. This chapter describes the process of psychotherapy that primarily focused on treating the relational aspects of the partnership that seemed to be contributing to a loss of sexual desire.

DOI: 10.4324/9781003265023-7

The development of object relations theory has led psychoanalytic therapists to think about sex with an "emphasis on the qualities of relatedness to the object" (Parsons, 2000), where practitioners "think about sex in terms of relating and relating in terms of sex" (Colman, 2009, p. 25). Thus, as Colman suggests, practitioners tend either to interpret towards sex, where interpersonal relating is explored in terms of metaphors of sex; or interpret away from sex, where the interpretive stance is geared to exploring the way in which actual sex reveals relational dynamics in metaphorical terms. This characteristic may be a feature of other psychoanalytic approaches, and it is with a review of some of these that I begin in order to provide some context.

## Theoretical backdrop

In psychotherapeutic work with adult couples, difficulties that arise within sexual relationships are generally explored using three dominant narratives. The attachment narrative looks at ways in which disturbed patterns of attachment to the primary caregiver in infancy might contribute to difficulties in adult sexual relations (Caruso, 2011). The Oedipal narrative examines how difficulties in negotiating the "Oedipus situation" (Klein, 1928) are a crucial precursor to the development of a capacity to form intimate adult couple relationships. The "claustro–agoraphobic" narrative, as described by Rey (1994), describes the dilemma where the individuals in close relationships feel caught between fears of engulfment and fears of abandonment (Balfour, 2005), a narrative that corresponds with autistic–contiguous anxieties (Berg, 2012).

### The attachment narrative

Bowlby's (1982) Attachment Theory, which described behaviour indicating an infant's love for and attachment to their caregivers, involves a correspondence between two distinct innate behavioural systems: attachment and caregiving. Shaver et al. (1988) extended Bowlby's theory to studying romantic love and adult couple relationships. They, and those following them who have taken account of sexuality in adult attachment, argue that when the attachment, caregiving, and sexual systems are functioning optimally, stable, and mutually satisfactory affectional bonds are formed and maintained, whereas malfunctioning "creates relational tensions, conflicts, dissatisfaction, and instability" (Mikulincer, 2006, p. 25).

Clulow and Boerma's (2009) observation, that patterns of attachment get enacted as dramas in the sexual arena, corroborates the growing empirical evidence that sexual dysfunction is a major source of relational conflict, that, according to Mikulincer, "can raise doubts about being loved and loving a partner, heighten worries and concerns about one's relationship ... and ultimately erode the affectional bond and destroy the relationship" (Mikulincer, 2006, p. 35). Clulow and Boerma propose that disorders of sexual desire might be considered as corresponding to insecure patterns of attachment, where couples who fear sexual desire in a loving relationship might seemingly desire sex but instead, "perpetuate a fusion in their relationship that kills off desire" (Clulow & Boerma, 2009, p. 88). They believe that such couples fear surrendering themselves to sexual intercourse because it "threatens to unleash uncontainable repressed feelings" (Clulow & Boerma, 2009, p. 89).

### The Oedipal narrative

Through an object relations lens, Grier (2005) looks at sexual difficulties as being part of an Oedipal narrative. He believes individuals erect rigid defences against knowing about the pain of feeling excluded from the primal scene of parents in intercourse. The avoidance of knowing about this reality is part of a universal tendency to "turn a blind eye to what we do not want to know" (Grier, 2005, p. 3) which, he believes, can lead to heterosexual adults developing serious relationship problems in the arena of sex.

Britton (1989), a post-Kleinian thinker, describes the importance of negotiating the Oedipal Situation and establishing a "third position" whereby one can know that one is excluded from the couple, and yet still know that one is loved by the parents. In this description, Britton illustrates the importance of developing the capacity for linked separateness, a third position in relation to the object. Failure to achieve this is associated by him with difficulties in sharing psychic space with another person, as though bringing two psychic realities together will have catastrophic consequences.

The Oedipal narrative, as well as the attachment narrative, is helpful in thinking about the absence of sex in intimate partnerships. However,

alone they do not sufficiently explain the absence of sex in couple relationships where the central conflict is one in which partners are struggling to maintain a strong sense of their own individual identity
alongside being part of a mutually satisfying couple relationship. For
this the "claustro–agoraphobic" narrative, as described by Rey (1994)
and Balfour (2005), is more helpful.

### The "claustro–agoraphobic" narrative

This narrative is a clinical description of adults caught in a relationship where intimacy generates feelings of claustrophobia and separateness or difference between the partners engenders feelings of
abandonment. Such anxieties hinder the development of satisfactory
intimate adult relationships and consequently present an important
area of consideration for clinicians working with couples presenting
sexual problems.

Glasser (1979) offers a contemporary Freudian perspective in
describing claustro–agoraphobic anxieties arising in the earliest relationship between infant and mother. He suggested that these kinds of
anxieties in adults relating arise from a "core complex" embedded
within the infant's most primitive relations with its mother. He
describes how the infant faces a conflict between an intense desire for
contact with mother, a wish to ultimately merge with her, and the fear
that such a merger will result in an annihilation of self. In response to
this "annihilation anxiety," the infant mobilises aggression in the service of self-preservation. This aggression is directed at the mother, and
the infant withdraws from the mother as a means of defending against
the threat of engulfment and subsequent obliteration. The consequent
withdrawal and wish to destroy the mother are then associated with
the converse fear, that of abandonment.

Glasser saw the "core complex" as being a pre-Oedipal phenomenon, one that belongs to the struggle within a two-person relationship
(i.e., mother and infant), from which fathers are absent, well predating
awareness of the relationship between parents when triangular
three-person dynamics come into play. He does not focus specifically
on the Oedipus complex because, for him, the Oedipus complex is
only an issue later on in development. But he suggests all Oedipal difficulties may stem from earlier problems associated with the "core
complex."

I shall focus on this third narrative, the "claustro–agoraphobic" narrative. I will explore how anxieties observable in psychotherapeutic work with couples can have their roots in the infant's earliest relations with the mother and can be traced back to Glasser's idea of the "core complex." I shall show how I have used this idea to inform my clinical work with two couples where a sexual relationship was desired by one partner but absent in the relationship. Both couples struggled with the "claustro–agoraphobic dilemma" –how to maintain a sense of self without feeling consumed by the relationship. I am indebted to the couples for consenting to material from their therapies being used in this chapter.

## The couples

Couple A sought help citing the lack of sex in their relationship as the presenting problem. Both partners jointly concurred that the problem lay in the husband's loss of desire. Mrs A was convinced that all the couples they knew had a good and regular sex life and felt deprived by this, whereas Mr A felt he could not have sex with Mrs A for all sorts of emotional reasons but primarily because the couple argued bitterly. He needed the arguments to stop, and for his wife to be less critical of him, in order to feel close to her.

Conversely, Couple B did not mention the absence of sex during their assessment interview. The issue gradually emerged as being one of many complaints that Mr B had about Mrs B, that she denied him sex. Like Mrs A, Mr B also felt entitled to a regular and satisfying sex life and was convinced that his wife was deliberately depriving him of physical contact. Mrs B, on the other hand, felt her husband needed to be less critical and diminishing of her before she could feel trusting and close to him.

### Couple A

Mr and Mrs A sought treatment because of Mr A's disinterest in sex. They had been together for several years, and for a brief period after they got together the couple had enjoyed good sex. However, shortly after their first argument with each other Mr A lost interest in sex. Since then, and over the many years that followed, Mrs A had tried a myriad of ways to revive Mr A's sexual interest in her but without much success. Interestingly, the couple had married after many years of living together, when sex had also been absent from their relationship.

Both partners in couple A describe a lonely childhood and shared early experiences of prolonged trauma, including maternal rejection and unpredictable separations. Mrs A was the only daughter of parents who are now deceased. Shortly after her birth, her mother had a breakdown and was hospitalised for nearly a year. During this first year, Mrs A was looked after in turns by relatives, all of whom she described as being "uninterested and useless" (although, of course, she would have no conscious memory of this time). She recalled growing up with a mother who seemed frequently distracted, giving her the experience of being with someone whose mind was not on her. Mr A grew up in a large family where he was the second child. He represented his mother as being absorbed in caring for his older, weaker brother at his expense, while being totally oblivious to his own desperate attempts to attract her attention. Mr A thought he received more beatings than his other siblings: he described his mother unfairly punishing him and then, upon his father's return home, complaining to his father, who would then beat him further. Mr A thought his parents had a poor relationship where they rowed regularly. He described an early memory of his father reaching for mother's hand during a family holiday; in response, his mother had recoiled and publicly berated his father. Mr and Mrs A's histories made me wonder whether unconsciously the couple might be united in their joint struggle in dealing with abandoning objects, and whether an unconscious desire for resolution might underlie the compulsive re-enactment of this dynamic between them. Mr and Mrs A's experiences of growing up with mothers who appeared impervious to their needs also made me wonder whether one of the couple's shared unconscious phantasies might be of a joint longing for fusion with the perfectly attuned mother. Over the course of therapy, we discovered that the partners shared an unconscious longing for fusion as a defence against separateness. For each partner, intimacy was associated with the fear of an inextricable merger with the other; yet separation stirred up unbearable feelings of abandonment.

## A clinical vignette

About six months into the work, the couple arrived at their session not speaking to each other. Mrs A sat upright in her seat. Her jaw was set as she looked directly at me. Mr A looked pale and lifeless, with dark rings under his eyes. He stared desolately into his lap. In a matter-of-fact, emotionless voice, Mrs A related how, at the weekend, she had suggested to her husband that they jointly plan their summer holiday, and Mr A had refused, saying it felt like work. An argument erupted. Mr A stormed off to his room (the couple were in separate bedrooms) and ended up not speaking to his wife for four days. During this time Mrs A felt distraught. She impressed upon me her conviction that, by being silent, her husband was punishing her. She said she was absolutely furious at being abandoned and left alone. Then she stopped speaking and stared directly at me, pinning me with her eyes, waiting for me to respond. Addressing Mrs A, I raised the possibility that Mr A might be struggling too. She scoffed at this and stated dismissively that she was fed up with trying to understand her husband. She had had enough and wanted out of the marriage. The session then slumped into silence.

In the silence, I began to track back internally on what had just transpired between us. Mrs A had begun by showing me how badly behaved Mr A had been and had possibly expected me to join her in criticising him. Perhaps she needed me to understand her despair at feeling abandoned by her husband at the weekend when she was proposing a shared activity. Instead, I responded unsympathetically to her, possibly leaving her feeling abandoned by me. It seemed as if unconsciously I had become very closely aligned, perhaps even psychically merged, with Mr A's experience of events while giving Mrs A the impression that she was in the presence of a misattuned therapist whose mind was not on her.

As the session progressed it emerged that Mr A had been feeling exhausted after a hard week at work with very little sleep; just the thought of doing anything at all at the weekend filled him with fatigue. He did not communicate this to Mrs A because he was convinced that she knew how he was feeling. This is why he felt incensed that she was being inconsiderate and selfish, so much so that he simply had to get away from her; hence he locked himself in his room. However, once he had calmed down, he began to feel frightened of rejoining her, apprehensive of what he might find, so he stayed in his room feeling miserable and alone.

In this session, I had not managed to attend to Mrs A's distress. In fact, during the first year of therapy I struggled to maintain an even-handed approach to the couple, finding it increasingly difficult not to take sides. It felt challenging to think about the partners as being part of a couple, and of what might be going on between them.

The persistence of my countertransference experience when work-ing with this couple, that is, being continually unconsciously tugged into re-enacting a two-person relationship in the room, led me to view this couple's interaction through the lens of the "core complex" (Glasser, 1979). When viewed from this perspective, it seemed plausible that a distraught Mrs A had come to the session nursing an intense unconscious craving for perfect understanding from me (mother/ther-apist). According to Glasser this kind of unconscious intensity can generate an "annihilation anxiety," and aggression is activated to pre-serve a sense of self. Perhaps Mrs A unconsciously feared that perfect understanding would result in the two of us becoming psychically merged, resulting in a loss of her own sense of self. Certainly, in the session, I had experienced Mrs A as being rather antagonistic towards me. My response was unsympathetic to her and this left her feeling abandoned and hopeless. This dynamic seemed similarly re-enacted between the partners at the weekend: Mr A appeared to nurture an unconscious belief that his wife should perfectly understand, and know, exactly how he was feeling. This illusion of psychic fusion func-tions as a defence against the reality of knowing there are two separate people in the marriage having different experiences. When Mr A's delu-sion was challenged by his wife's request to help her plan their holiday, rather than intuitively know he was feeling absolutely exhausted and wanted to be left alone to rest, he responded aggressively and withdrew to his room. Withdrawal might also be unconsciously designed to pro-tect his wife from the force of the aggression he felt towards her. His fear of rejoining her might be understood, then, as an indicator of the strength of the aggression he felt towards her, and of his anxiety about confronting the damage he had unconsciously inflicted upon her.

Three years into the clinical work the strength of the projective sys-tem slowly began to loosen. The couple gradually began to bring evi-dence of an increase in their joint capacity to be reflective and to think about themselves, and of themselves as being part of a couple. This coincided with a shift in my countertransference when I began to feel I had a couple in the room. There seemed to be more space to think and to be curious, and I felt able to attend to one partner without fearing I was excluding the other or that I was taking sides. This was evidenced by the couple's ability to tolerate my attention on one part-ner while simultaneously remaining engaged and curious about what they might discover about the other.

By the time the therapy ended, the partners had managed to have penetrative sex, which they both found deeply satisfying. They had become more actively engaged with knowing about their own, and each other's emotional experience, and were better able to come together and comfort each other, and also to think together about themselves in relation to each other. As they left therapy, they expressed their wish to continue working towards creating and sustaining a more gratifying relationship which had developed between them.

## Couple B

Mr and Mrs B had been married for over thirty years. Mr B was a retired professional whereas Mrs B continued working at a more leisurely pace. At the point the couple sought help, they were barely speaking to each other. Mr B complained bitterly about his wife's total lack of interest in him or in their marriage. Mrs B had a defeated air about her and she attributed her weariness to years of irresolvable, circuitous arguments in which she had felt unheard and trampled on by her husband. To engage with Mr B, she felt, would mean succumbing to a loss of her individuality and to becoming an extension of him – the image of what he wanted her to be. Therefore, she felt it was safer to withdraw into herself than to engage with him. Her withdrawal frustrated and infuriated Mr B, who responded by flying into rages about feeling neglected and abandoned by her.

Each partner shared early experiences of maternal deprivation. Mr B described his mother as cold, hard, cruel, and rejecting, and presented us with examples of how his father's attempts to comfort and care for him did not, in any way, compensate for his intense longing for mother's attention and love, which he felt he never received. Mrs B, on the other hand, described her father as harsh and punishing, disparaging of her and belittling her abilities. She described her mother as being unprotective and critical of her, and of complaining unrelentingly about her efforts to care for her in her later years when she became infirm. The couple's histories provided some evidence for believing that they might be united in their shared longing for an attuned and responsive maternal object, but they protected themselves through becoming locked into recreating a more familiar relationship with the critical, disappointing, and abusive parental object.

The couple had sought couple therapy twice before. In both instances they had abandoned therapy because they felt utterly convinced that the therapist had formed an alliance with one of them against the other, making the excluded partner the "problem" in the room. Hence, at the assessment stage it was thought Couple B might benefit from being seen in co-therapy, which is how they were seen.

At the start of therapy, Mr B brought his wife as the problem to be resolved, but as time went on he became concerned that the therapists were allying themselves with his wife, making him the focus of attention but also the problem. As the therapy progressed he began to align himself with the male therapist; he expressed how similar he was to my colleague and his belief that they were of similar ages. That they wore similar shoes was simply more evidence of their shared connection. However, Mr B viewed me, the female therapist, with suspicion, as he felt I was very similar to his wife. This view of me was further strengthened by his observation that Mrs B and I frequently dressed in similar coloured clothing, and therefore he felt justified in relating to me as if she and I were the same. My countertransference, during this early phase of therapy was primarily one where I felt drawn into an identification with Mrs B's experience of being at the receiving end of Mr B's aggressive and unreasonable behaviour. Also, in my countertransference, I sometimes felt anxious about expressing a thought that was different to Mr B's as it had the potential for escalating into an argument rather than an exploration. So strong could this be that at times I feared that if I ventured into an area that he did not wish to explore he might, in fury, simply refuse to attend the sessions and abandon the therapy altogether. I did not take this anxiety up with Mr B, but Mrs B said how hugely relieved she had felt when she witnessed her husband being intransigent with me and unavailable to consider another point of view. She felt this was exactly how he was with her at home.

As the therapy developed, Mr B's use of idealisation as a defence against relating began to come to the fore. In the consulting room, he would frequently conjure up images of happy summer holidays that the couple could enjoy if only things were different between them. However, his unrealised dreams became a justification for his catalogue of complaints against Mrs B, that she would not play the part that would sustain this ideal image, and additionally, that she refused him sex. Mrs B's pivotal anxiety, that she unreservedly expressed, was that if she were to recognise or respond to Mr B's "bottomless" needs, or indeed have sex with him at all, it would open the floodgates, leaving her totally overwhelmed and diminished in relation to him. So, between them I observed them managing their respective anxieties about having a closer relationship through regulating the emotional and, more concretely, the physical distance between them. Although they lived together, they would inhabit and retreat to different parts of their house where the other was not welcome.

The following clinical vignette illustrates a dominant theme in Couple B's therapy: both partners harbouring high hopes of an idealised relationship but being relentlessly exposed to the crashing disappointment of how they actually interacted with each other. It captures how an idealised image of reunion is shattered by deep disillusionment of coming together when the reality of a differentiated other explodes the fantasy of slotting neatly into the internal world image.

### A clinical vignette

About eighteen months into therapy Mr B arrived for the session feeling so angry that he could not speak, leaving Mrs B to explain the series of events that had led to this scenario. She said that Mr B had been away for a few days, holidaying with a close friend, and had been unclear about his return plans. However, on the day he was to return home he had telephoned her with an estimated time of arrival. She said she had wanted to be home to welcome Mr B, but around the time he was due back she had been unexpectedly called away from home to rescue a stranded friend who had telephoned her for help. As Mrs B walked back home after successfully helping her friend, she began to feel anxious about not having been able to welcome Mr B back. On opening the front door, she said she found Mr B sitting on the stairs like a little boy lost. He had begun to tell her that he had a migraine and that his head hurt at which she had become alarmed, and this must have shown on her face. Mr B then complained that she had "made the wrong face," and had refused to speak to her since.

Prompted to describe his experience, Mr B said that they had been feeling close when he had left for his holiday. He confirmed Mrs B's account of events upon his coming home, but added that he had been tired because he had travelled a long distance and making his way back during the rush hour on public transport had given him a head-ache. He had been looking forward to seeing Mrs B, and when he had not found her at home he had proceeded to deposit his bags in his bedroom. As he was coming back downstairs, he heard her key in the lock. He sat on the stairs in a "jolly fashion" waiting to greet her as she walked through the door. The look he had seen on Mrs B's face conveyed to him that she was horrified and disappointed at his return, and not joyously welcoming of him as he had hoped. Mr B simply could not get over this crushing blow. He had refused to entertain Mrs B's experience of the incident and had remained angry about Mrs B's rejection of him. This reaction to her having "made the wrong face," had lasted for days until they came for therapy.

In the session we explored the possibility that Mr B may have experienced Mrs B's alarm, a response to her anxiety about her husband's health, as if she were a rejecting, unsympathetic mother unable to contain his distress and comfort him. Mr B saw the parallel but remained unconvinced that this might have influenced his reaction towards his wife. In contrast, Mrs B seemed more able to consider her maternal transference response towards Mr B in this episode, when he had behaved like the demanding and emotionally depleting mother who had made her feel resentfully responsible for her well-being.

Two years into the therapy, the projective system between the partners seemed to have relaxed: both partners increasingly reported that they were getting on better, that things felt calmer between them and that there were fewer heated arguments at home. Around this time, I began to notice a modification in the quality of my countertransference response to the couple, where I felt more aligned with Mr B's painful struggle in the face of Mrs B's deliberate unavailability to him. This coincided with a shift in Mrs B's emotional state, where her presentation began to alter from being the more emotionally available partner to being more assertive, particularly in response to challenges about her part in perpetrating the difficulties between them. The therapy ended with both partners saying they recovered more quickly from arguments, that were noticeably less pernicious, and although they had not reached the point where they could have sex, this was being entertained as a prospect.

## Discussion

A significant feature of therapy with Couple A and Couple B, particularly in the first year of treatment, was that the partners in both couples seemed to be caught up in unconsciously recreating two-person relationships in which themes of a longing to merge and fuse with an other seemed to dominate. This was enacted in the therapy, too, where there seemed to be a strong pull to recreate two-person relationships within the clinical setting. This was evidenced by my countertransference response in both cases where I found myself engaged in a therapeutic struggle to maintain an even-handed approach towards the partners. For example, in Couple A, I now think Mr A unconsciously engineered a two-person interaction in the room as a defence against separateness and difference. He rendered himself non-existent by psychically hiding behind Mrs A, while the exchanges between Mrs A and I became quite heated. Conversely, by psychically aligning himself with me and dispensing with differences of opinion, it felt as if Mr A and I were getting along comfortably. Here, Mrs A became the "problem" in the room that Mr A unconsciously offered to me for "fixing." This felt similar to Mrs A overtly naming Mr A as the problem and bringing him to therapy for, as she termed it, "sorting out."

In Couple B the roles were reversed: Mrs B presented as having been the long suffering wife of a belligerent and unreasonable husband who simply criticised and berated her seemingly unprovoked. In the room, she often became non-existent, psychically hiding behind her husband who effortlessly took up most of the space in the room with his complaints about his wife's withholding behaviour. Initially, when I attempted to challenge Mr B's overt denigration of Mrs B in the room, the interaction between Mr B and I could become agitated and tense. At these points Mrs B seemed to psychically align herself with me; she would remain silent but glance at me helplessly, as if in empathic recognition. In countertransference terms, I felt inseparably identified with her experience of relating to an impossible and unreasonable man. Furthermore, as the therapy progressed, my co-therapist and I could find ourselves taking up positions that were divided along gender lines: my co-therapist could find himself feeling identified with Mr B's vulnerability and experience Mrs B's silent provocation. Similarly, I could become identified with Mrs B's experience of being ruthlessly denigrated by her husband. Once again, in the room, it seemed as if only two-person relationships could exist. There was a noteworthy absence of a third.

The unconscious enactment of merging psychically with an other can be thought about as a defence against the psychic pain that separation entails, and also the pain of knowing that one is separate from the object of one's desire and therefore unable to control it. The re-enactment of this dynamic, through attempts to create exclusive, merged pairs or divided hostile ones, made me wonder whether, for both couples, something quite primitive, possibly belonging to the mother–infant dyad, might be operational, where the presence of a third seemed strikingly absent. This signalled the possibility that Glasser's concept of the "core complex" might form part of both couples' shared unconscious phantasy.

Another common feature between the therapies of these couples was their difficulty in committing to the therapy. For Couple A, after each argument that the couple had at home, one or other of the partners would threaten divorce and express a wish to end therapy. Often after an argument, Mr A would not attend a session and Mrs A would come alone, wishing to settle the account and terminate therapy. At each of these points I would write to Mr A inviting him back, which he accepted, and the subsequent sessions would take on a very tentative feel in which I would work cautiously to reengage the couple. In the case of Couple B, Mr B frequently expressed a wish to be free of the weekly commitment to therapy, stating it curtailed his freedom to travel at will. Mrs B remained reserved about expressing what she wanted and, although she claimed the therapy was helping her in finding her voice in the relationship, the therapists got a sense that she would go along with whatever Mr B wanted. This oscillation –where ongoing therapy might be terminated at short notice –was very unsettling for the therapists. In the countertransference, we felt as if we were walking on eggshells with Mr B who might abandon us by abruptly stopping coming. In therapy with both couples, the overall countertransference experience was one of oscillating between being lulled into a sense of feeling settled in the therapeutic work, and suddenly, and often unexpectedly, being faced with the threat of an abrupt ending. Over time, I came to understand this oscillation between the wish for sublime merger and the sudden threat of abandonment as a feature of the "core complex" phenomenon.

A further theme running through the therapy of both couples, and one that added to the complexity of treatment, was that it felt impossible to speak openly about sex in the consulting room. Right at the start of therapy Mr A thwarted my attempts to talk about sex openly by stating very plainly that he did not want to talk about sex in the sessions, and that if I persisted he would stop coming. This posed a working dilemma: on the one hand, how could we address the presenting problem for which the couple had sought help when Mr A refused to talk about sex; on the other, how might Mrs A's increasingly resentful feeling that not only was her husband denying her sex but was now also refusing to talk about it in therapy be engaged? As she put it: "I always have to go along with what you want. What about what I want? What about me?"

In Couple B's case, Mr B's insistence that Mrs B should have sex with him to show him that she cared for him fell on deaf ears. Mrs B refused to entertain this idea, let alone discuss it in the consulting room, as she felt that he had disregarded all the other ways she showed her affection towards him. In addition, she felt that to have sex with Mr B would mean she were succumbing to his demands, where she existed only in relation to pleasing him and not as a person in her own right. She felt that to preserve her sanity and her own sense of self she needed to resist his sexual demands. Convinced of this, she refused to entertain any further exploration of the issue in the room.

To talk about sex openly in the room with either couple would have meant that Mr A as well as Mrs B would have felt discounted and abandoned the therapy. But not to talk about it risked discounting Mrs A and Mr B. This dilemma signalled to me that part of the couples' shared unconscious phantasy revolved around the "core complex" theme, namely the phantasy that intimacy can only be achieved at the expense of one or other partner and therefore needs avoiding at all costs.

The technical dilemma resulting from this places in a new light Colman's (2009) choice between interpreting towards or away from sexual content in the material. Drawing on the "core complex" concept implies a stance that interprets away from sex and towards the anxieties associated with intimacy and the threat of abandonment. But to adopt that stance in couple work can risk surrendering therapeutic balance. In countertransference terms, it may be experienced as an extreme version of being torn by the pull of forming a collusive alliance with one partner against the other. The technical challenge is to maintain a space in which such either/or resolutions can be thought about and transformed into a reflective capacity that contains the anxiety associated with each of the poles and enabling a third position to be found: in developmental terms, moving from a pre- Oedipal to Oedipal state of mind.

## Conclusion

In this chapter, I have described aspects of therapy with two couples where the unconscious fear of merger or abandonment resulted in behaviour that unconsciously regulated the emotional distance between the partners. Oscillating between the fear of merger and the threat of abandonment, they each avoided their feared catastrophe by either killing off the potential for connection between them or by capitulating in order not to be abandoned.

This theme of merger vs. abandonment could also be tracked through my countertransference experience where, in the initial stages of working with both couples, there were times when I felt unable to think in the room with them, to hold on to my own perspective without imposing it on them. I struggled with this countertransference experience of becoming overwhelmed to the extent that my own reflective capacities became affected, as it signalled a collapse of the difference in our respective positions within the consulting room. The obliteration of difference not only posed a threat to the couple, but also to the therapy. The torn countertransference response can be a clinical indicator of pre-Oedipal themes which are best understood in terms of the "core complex," and which can then be played out in that most intimate of couple domains – their sexual relationship.

Interestingly, Glasser's concept carries the implication that clinicians will interpret away from sex to the underlying dynamics around anxiety about survival of the self. Such a therapeutic stance can recreate the root of the problem for partners like Mrs A and Mr B, whose framing of the problem of emotional deprivation in terms of lack of sex in the relationship then gets disregarded. Equally, the problem is restated if sex becomes the focus of work, where the existential threat is picked up by partners such as Mr A and Mrs B. In these circumstances therapists are challenged both to immerse themselves in and free themselves of the technical bind in which they find themselves, a bind that restates the developmental problem for which help is being sought. The experience can be one of emotional oscillation, and it is in containing the anxieties associated with intimacy and autonomy that progress can be made.

# References

American Psychiatric Association. (2013). *Diagnostic and statistical manual of mental disorders* (5th ed.). https://doi.org/10.1176/appi.books.9780890425596

Balfour, A. (2005). The couple, their marriage, and Oedipus: or, problems come in twos and threes. In: F. Grier (Ed.), *Oedipus and the couple* (pp. 49–72). London: Karnac.

Berg, J. (2012) "A bad moment with the light." No-sex couples: the role of autistic-contiguous anxieties. *Couple and Family Psychoanalysis*, 2(1), 33–48.

Bowlby, J. (1982). *Attachment and loss: Vol. 1: Attachment* (2nd edn). New York: Basic Books [original edition published 1969].

Britton, R. (1989). The missing link: parental sexuality in the Oedipus complex. In: J. Steiner (Ed.), *The Oedipus complex today: Clinical implications* (pp. 83–101). London: Karnac.

Caruso, N. (2011). The entangled nature of attachment and sexuality in the couple relationship. *Couple and Family Psychoanalysis*, 1(1), 117–135.

Clulow, C., & Boerma, M. (2009). Dynamics and disorders of sexual desire. In: C. Clulow (Ed.), *Sex, attachment and couple psychotherapy: Psychoanalytic perspectives* (pp. 75–102). London: Karnac.

Colman, W. (2009). What do we mean by "sex"? In: C. Clulow (Ed.), *Sex, attachment and couple psychotherapy: Psychoanalytic perspectives* (pp. 25–44). London: Karnac.

Glasser, M. (1979). Some aspects of the role of aggression in the perversions. In: I. Rosen (Ed.), *Sexual Deviation* (2nd edn, pp. 278–305). Oxford: Oxford University Press.

Green, L., & Seymour, J. (2009). Loss of desire: a psycho-sexual case study. In: C. Clulow (Ed.), *Sex, attachment and couple psychotherapy: Psychoanalytic perspectives* (pp. 141–164). London: Karnac.

Grier, F. (2005). *Oedipus and the couple*. London: Karnac.

Klein, M. (1928). Early stages of the Oedipus conflict. *International Journal of Psycho-Analysis*, 9, 167–180 [reprinted in *Love, Guilt and Reparation*]. London: Hogarth, 1975.

Mikulincer, M. (2006). Attachment, caregiving and sex within romantic relationships: a behavioral systems perspective. In: M. Mikulincer & G. Goodman (Eds.), *Dynamics of romantic love: Attachment, caregiving and sex* (pp. 23–44). New York & London: Guilford.

Parsons, M. (2000). Sexuality and perversion a hundred years on: discovering what Freud discovered. *International Journal of Psycho-Analysis*, 81, 37–49.

Rey, H. (1994). *Universals of psychoanalysis in the treatment borderline states*. London: Free Association.

Shaver, P. R., Hazan, C., & Bradshaw, D. (1988). Love as attachment: the integration of three behavioural systems. In: R. J. Sternberg & L. Michael (Eds.), *Psychology of love* (pp. 68–99). New Haven, CT: Yale University Press.

# Chapter 8

# Discussion of "Viewing the absence of sex from couple relationships through the 'core complex' lens"

*James Poulton*

Amita Sehgal's chapter, "Viewing the absence of sex from couple relationships through the 'core complex' lens," exhibits the characteristics that have become a hallmark of her writing: a philosopher's appreciation of the complexities involved in couple interactions; a deep familiarity with analytic theory and practice; and an acute sensitivity to the subtly nuanced relationships that comprise couple psychotherapy. In this paper, Sehgal has turned her powers of observation to couples experiencing sexual difficulties and to the primitive intrapsychic and interactive dynamics underlying them. She begins by stating that these difficulties are generally explored via "three dominant narratives": the attachment narrative, which links such difficulties to insecure attachment patterns and unconscious efforts by the couple to "kill off" fear-inducing sexual desire; the Oedipal narrative, according to which partners fear sharing psychic space and "erect rigid defences against knowing the pain of feeling excluded from the primal scene"; and the "claustro-agoraphobic" narrative, which suggests these difficulties are derived from pre-Oedipal dynamics in the infant-mother relationship.

Sehgal tells us that, in working with two couples in which a sexual relationship was desired by one partner but rejected by the other, she found that this third narrative was most helpful in conceptualising and working through the couples' difficulties. Specifically, she states that because both couples experienced claustrophobic anxieties in moments of intimacy and fears of abandonment when separate, she viewed them as exhibiting the dynamics of Glasser's (1979) "core complex," which essentially describes an infant caught in a paralysing middle ground between desiring and fearing both closeness with its mother (threatening engulfment and annihilation of the infant's self), and separateness from her (threatening abandonment and loss).

DOI: 10.4324/9781003265023-8

Sehgal states that this narrative excludes the father, since it "belongs to the struggle within a two-person relationship (i.e., mother and infant), from which fathers are absent, well pre-dating awareness of the relationship between parents when triangular three-person dynamics come into play" (this volume, p. 87). The core complex, it seems, when applied to adult sexual difficulties, reaffirms the poetic wisdom in Royston's statement that "sexuality ... is infancy in a new erotic form, babyhood in a different jacket" (2001, p. 37).

The exclusion of the father in core complex theory seems to me to introduce problematic considerations from both theoretical and clinical perspectives. From a clinical viewpoint, as I read through Sehgal's case descriptions, particularly including the partners' childhood experiences, I find that *other* interpretations of their interactions, which refer to both mother and father and to triangulated relationships, keep presenting themselves as possibilities. And from a theoretical viewpoint, the "infinite" nature of "mental space" (Bion, 1970, p. 14) seems to me to argue against the possibility that any behaviour or experience – whether intrapsychic or interactive – is dominated solely by structural relationships stemming from a single developmental phase.

These considerations lead me to suspect that the difficulties exhibited by Sehgal's couples may be linked to at least three other theoretical arenas, all interrelated and all connected, at least potentially, to the dynamics of the core complex via developmental, defensive, or regressive means. These three arenas include: (1) each individual's negotiation of the Oedipal conflict (already mentioned by Sehgal, but overlooked in favour of the core complex); (2) each individual's "internal couple" (i.e., their internalised representations of the expected ways in which couples function and operate), typically based in experiences with the original parental couple; and (3) the couple's *shared* internal couple, co-constructed from each partner's internal object relationships and containing a variety of shared phantasies, anxieties, and defences, as well as a joint ego, superego, and ego ideal, by which the couple unconsciously determines which behaviours "fit" their shared picture, and which do not. My purpose in introducing these dimensions is not to suggest that they would replace the explanations given by Sehgal, but rather that they might coexist with the dynamics of the core complex, and thereby enrich our understanding both of that complex and of the couples themselves. To illustrate how these dimensions may be integrated into the clinical picture Sehgal presents,

I'll now turn to one of the couples she describes, Mr and Mrs A, though I believe that my observations may be analogously applicable to her other couple.

Before we begin, a word about my method: Some of the observations that follow are the result of my own reveries as I have reflected upon the clinical material provided. As reveries, I cannot firmly demonstrate their validity, but, as clinicians know, such reveries have value as a potential means of generating hypotheses and exploring new dimensions that may illuminate heretofore hidden regions in the treatment of such couples. I am grateful that the insights and clarity of thought provided by Sehgal have created the fertile field in which such explorations can occur.

## Mr and Mrs A

Sehgal tells us that this couple sought treatment because of Mr A's disinterest in sex. The couple had been together for several years, and although they reported good sex at first, Mr A lost interest shortly after their first argument. Thereafter, Mrs A tried to revive their sexual relationship but found little success. Sehgal reports that both partners described a "lonely childhood and shared early experiences of prolonged trauma, including maternal rejection and unpredictable separations" (this volume, p. 89) Shortly after her birth, Mrs A's mother had a breakdown and was hospitalised for a year, during which Mrs A was looked after by "uninterested and useless" relatives. Once reunited, Mrs A found her mother to be "frequently distracted, giving her the experience of being with someone whose mind was not on her" (this volume, p. 90). Similarly, Mr A characterised his mother as being so absorbed in caring for his "weaker" older brother that she was oblivious to his attempts to attract her attention. He felt unfairly punished by his mother, who not only beat him, but complained to his father who, upon returning home, would beat him further. Mr A's parents fought frequently, and he reported an "early memory of his father reaching for mother's hand during a family holiday; in response, his mother had recoiled and publicly berated his father" (this volume, p. 89).

Sehgal states that Mr and Mrs A's histories made her "wonder whether unconsciously the couple might be united in their joint struggle in dealing with abandoning objects," (this volume, p. 89). and her report that treatment ultimately demonstrated the applicability of the core complex to this couple is convincing. I suspect, however, that the partners' unconscious internal representations of couples (their internal couples), were steeped in Oedipal issues, and this also played a role.

Psychoanalytic literature has linked the formation of an individual's internal couple to the dynamics of the Oedipal conflict. Klein (1945) linked the ambivalent emotions of the early stages of Oedipus to the infant's varying part-object and whole-object representations of the parents and their genitals, as well as the relationships between them. Klein suggested, for example, that by the middle of the first year the infant's oral desires are "transferred from the mother's breast to the father's penis," leading to envy and jealousy of the mother because she "receives this desired object" (the father's penis) to the exclusion of the infant (p. 78). Following Klein, Kernberg (1995) stated that as a mother leaves her infant "to return as a sexual woman to father," the infant identifies "with the sexual couple – that is, father as mother's object," which in turn "consolidates the triangular situation in the child's unconscious fantasy (pp. 29–30)." Similarly, Frisch and Frisch-Desmarez (2010) used Klein's concept of the "combined parents," which represents an early and persecutory fantasy that the "parents or their genital organs are inseparably united in a permanent sexual relationship" (p. 333), to suggest that even the most primitive image of the parental couple mobilises feelings of sexual exclusion. Only once the infant has successfully negotiated Oedipus, and has acquired a capacity for a "third position" (Britton, 1989) – through which the child masters the anxieties of being excluded (or of being part of a couple that excludes) and resolves ambivalent feelings of love and hate towards both parents – that a less persecutory internal couple becomes established (Fisher, 1993; Rosenthall, 2007). Morgan and Freedman (2000) succinctly summarise this relationship between Oedipus and the internal couple: a "healthy resolution of the Oedipus complex results in the introjection of the kind of internal object that we might describe as an internal creative couple" (see also Morgan, 2005), while disruptions of the Oedipus complex "can result in disturbed internal couples that give rise to dysfunctional, and maybe even perverse, intimate relationships" (p. 86).

The childhood histories of Mr and Mrs A allow for a few educated guesses about their management of the Oedipal Situation and the consequent characteristics of their internal couples. Because of Mr A's past experiences, for example, we might imagine that his internal couple would contain a rejecting, contemptuous, and disinterested mother in a repetitive and conflicted relationship with a desiring, rejected, and violent father. If we accept this as a possible description of his internal couple, then a fairly straight line could be drawn between it and Mr A's anxious and self-protective withdrawal from his wife's (mother's) anger; his passive-aggressive attacks on her; his refusal to help plan a holiday (a re-enactment of the parental holiday event?); his subsequent four-day silence (another retreat from parental violence); and even his transference towards treatment. Mr A's failure to appear for sessions, as well as his rendering himself "non-existent by psychically hiding behind Mrs A" (this volume, p. 98) during periodic heated exchanges between Mrs A and Sehgal, can be seen as constituting the new, frightening parental couple.

Even more may be gleaned from Mr A's childhood once we examine it through the specific lens of an unresolved Oedipal struggle. Not only do his experiences describe a parental couple who offer neither succour nor compassion, and instead present an impenetrable front of aggression to the excluded child, but they also describe a couple in whom sexuality (symbolised by the father's attempt to hold the mother's hand) is rejected in a sadistic and castrating manner. Such experiences may have triggered castration anxieties in Mr A himself, and may have subsequently evolved into both a general expectation of what happens to sexuality once a couple is formed, and a specific expectation of what will happen to *him* if he attempts to be sexual. In this case, we might say that Mr A's failure to negotiate the Oedipal struggle created an internal couple that provokes paranoid anxieties, with accompanying unresolved longing and hatred for his (parental) persecutors. Such an internal couple would then be easily linked to his fear of sexuality with Mrs A, his aggression towards her around sexual issues, and his hypersensitivity to the conditions under which sex can occur.

Mrs A's childhood history allows us to make similar guesses about her negotiation with Oedipus and her internal couple. Sehgal's description of Mrs A's childhood doesn't mention Mrs A's father at all. Instead, we are told that during her first year, Mrs A stayed with relatives and thereafter lived with her "distracted" mother. We certainly *might* interpret the absence of the father in Sehgal's narrative as implying that he played little role in the formation of Mrs A's psyche. But a more likely interpretation is that a *missing father* (i.e., a figure who is supposed to be there, but who is instead "present in his absence" – Ruszczynski, 2020) was a significant figure in Mrs A's development.

From this perspective, we can also then identify several aspects of Mrs A's behaviour that can be linked to the missing father, either as a stand-alone figure or as half of an internal couple.

First, Sehgal tells us that Mrs A was furious at being "abandoned and left alone" after Mr A refused to help plan their vacation. In her fury, Mrs A "scoffed" at the possibility that Mr A might be struggling too and "stated dismissively that she was fed-up with trying to understand her husband" (this volume, p. 90). In my view, an act such as this, in which one person erases the internal world of another, is commonly accomplished via the projection of a persecutory internal figure (around which such polarised emotions as hate or fear revolve), which is then omnipotently assumed to represent the sole and absolute truth about the projection's recipient. But which figure is Mrs A projecting? Her mother? Perhaps. But might it also be her missing father, for whom Mrs A may have harboured deep resentment because he abandoned her? Second, we noted above that Mr A would attempt to "render himself non-existent" by hiding behind his wife, and Sehgal additionally tells us that after Mr and Mrs A argued at home, Mrs A would sometimes appear for therapy alone, asking to settle accounts and terminate treatment. It is possible to view these patterns as representing a re-enactment of Mrs A's experiences with her parents, effected through a dominating projective identification of her internal couple, and consisting of a dissatisfied, disinterested but present mother, and an abandoning and missing father. Third, Sehgal tells us that Mrs A exhibited transferential antagonism towards her after Sehgal noted that Mr A might be struggling. Sehgal suggests that this antagonism arises from Mrs A's fear that understanding from the therapist would result in merger and loss of self. But might not Mrs A's internal couple also be involved? Her anger towards Sehgal may have been rooted in a fear that Sehgal, as a stand-in mother, would fail to retrieve the missing father/husband, rendering her forever consigned to the persecutions of a disinterested and unsympathetic mother.

Mrs A's internal couple, as I have so far described it, is not one that would have been amenable to a successful resolution of the Oedipus complex. If, as O'Shaughnessy (1964) has stated, the absent object is a persecutory object, then both the mother and father in Mrs A's internal couple would have been felt to be irremediably threatening. These anxieties, coupled with the likelihood that Mrs A did not experience her parents as a real, functioning couple, leads me to suspect that she, like Mr A, had been unable to negotiate the difficulties of triangulated relationships. This left Mrs A. unable to integrate the polarised emotions that would have dominated her external and internal relationships with the parental couple. In such a case, I wonder whether, despite her protestations, Mrs A did not see sexual relations with her husband as unambiguously positive, but rather as a source of unconscious anxiety. If this interpretation is valid, then perhaps Mr A's avoidance of sexuality did not only originate in his own Oedipally related anxieties, but in Mrs A's as well.

This last point refers to the possibility that a shared internal couple – one that contained both partners' unresolved Oedipal phantasies, fears, and aggressions, and created over years of mutual projective and introjective identifications – was operating in the couple interactions and in their relationship with Sehgal. Such a shared internal couple would have included at least a frightening wife/mother who exhibited either disregard or castrating anger; a frightening husband/father who was either absent or actively violent; a shared phantasy that both could deliver intolerable losses and exclusions; and a shared "unconscious belief" (an unshakeable and self-limiting paranoid conviction) (Morgan, 2019) that generative, gratifying sexuality is an impossibility. All these aspects contributed to the partner's shared emotional stance of alternating longing and hatred. A shared internal couple such as this would have substantially impacted the development of the couple's shared unconscious and in turn would have effectuated specific aspects of their behaviour. The arguments between Mr and Mrs A, for example, that lead to threats of divorce and a wish to end therapy, could be interpreted as an enactment of the primary dilemmas of their shared internal couple. The couple's subsequent hesitance to re-engage in treatment could be viewed, first, as an expression of their unconscious certainty that there are no means available by which couples can amicably solve conflicts, and second, as a repetition of the defences they hold in common against such insoluble problems: a regressive reversion to aggression, infantile demand, and withdrawal.

## Can Oedipus, the internal couple (individual and shared), and the core complex coexist?

The essence of my view is that the possible presence of additional dimensions in Mr and Mrs A's relationship do not negate the insightful observations Sehgal makes about the permeating influence of the core complex. Rather, I see these dimensions as engaged in dialectical interactions with core complex dynamics, so that the couple's patterns are the result of contributions from each dimension. This perspective – that multiple dimensions or modes of psychic organisation may interact – has a long tradition in psychoanalytic theory. Ogden (1989), for example, described the autistic-contiguous position as standing in both a diachronic and a synchronic relationship to the paranoid-schizoid and depressive positions. Waddell (2002) stated that "there is a constant interplay … between the states of mind which generally characterize each developmental phase" (p. 8). More relevant to the difficulties presented by Mr and Mrs A, Guntrip (1962) suggested that the wish to regress to pre-Oedipal infantile dependence (an essential aspect of the core complex) is typically found in relation to failures in negotiating the Oedipus complex, which "stands midway between, and is a compromise between, infantile dependence in its ultimate form of regression and the maintenance of an active ego in real life" (p. 111).

As stated earlier, I believe that the specific mechanisms by which these multiple dimensions interact are either developmental, defensive, or regressive. If we were to attempt an integrated explanation of Mr and Mrs A's relationship using these dimensions, the following picture might emerge. Each partner, in their infancy, experienced an ambivalent relationship with a distracted or indifferent mother, leading them into the dynamics of the core complex. The unresolved nature of this complex, in coordination with the actual nature of the triangulated relationships within the family, then exerted a substantial developmental influence over the means available to them to negotiate the Oedipal Situation – leading them to not feel comfortable gravitating towards mother, father, nor the parental couple as a source of security and place. As they grew into adulthood, the anxieties, phantasies, and polarised emotions embedded in these multiple dimensions emerged in their relationship, instigating enactments both of parental malfunction and of Oedipal dramas. In defence against the more frightening aspects of these conflicts, each partner attempted to establish a bulwark of safety via a regressive retreat to the dyadic relationship with a wished-for mother. However, since the only mother available was the mother of the core complex, their retreat was an ineffective defence because it, too, exposed them to dangers – of intrusion, fusion, abandonment, and loss of self, all so well explicated by Sehgal.

## Conclusion

In this discussion, I have proposed, based on theoretical and clinical considerations, a broadening of our conceptualisation of the potential factors involved when a couple experiences difficulties in intimate relationships. This broader perspective allows for the possibility that the couple may exhibit core complex dynamics, but not as a stand-alone disturbance. Rather, the couple's difficulties can be seen as arising from the dialectical interaction between multiple dimensions, each hailing from differing developmental and relational phases. In Mr and Mrs A's case, the clinical material suggests that the obstacles in their intimate relationship were linked to their use of the core complex as a defensive retreat from unresolved conflicts related both to the Oedipal struggle and to the many painful experiences that formed their individual and shared internal couples. The fact that such a retreat failed to provide security for Mr and Mrs A, and instead created additional anxieties, only underscores the poignancy of the multiple dilemmas they were facing.

## References

Bion, W. R. (1970). *Attention and interpretation.* London: Tavistock Publications.

Britton, R. (1989). The missing link: Parental sexuality in the Oedipus complex. In J. Steiner (Ed.), *The Oedipus complex today: Clinical implications* (pp. 83–102). London: Karnac.

Fisher, J. (1993). The impenetrable other: Ambivalence and the Oedipal conflict in work with couples. In S. Ruszczynski (Ed.), *Psychotherapy with couples: Theory and practice at the Tavistock Institute of marital studies* (pp. 142–166). London: Karnac.

Frisch, S. and Frisch-Desmarez, C. (2010). Some thoughts on the concept of the internal parental couple. *International Journal of Psycho-Analysis*, 91(2): 325–342.

Glasser, M. (1979). Some aspects of the role of aggression in the perversions. In I. Rosen (Ed.), *Sexual deviation* (2nd Ed., pp. 278–305). Oxford: Oxford University Press.

Guntrip, H. (1962). The manic-depressive problem in the light of the schizoid process. *International Journal of Psycho-Analysis*, 43: 98–112.

Kernberg, O. F. (1995). *Love relations: Normality and pathology.* New Haven, CT: Yale University Press.

Klein, M. (1945). The Oedipus complex in the light of early anxieties. In R. Money-Kyrle (Ed.), *The writings of Melanie Klein, Vol. 1, Love, guilt and reparation and other works 1921–1945* (pp. 370–419). New York: Free Press, 1975.

Morgan, M. (2019). *A couple state of mind: Psychoanalysis of couples and the Tavistock relationships model.* Milton Park and New York: Routledge.

Morgan, M. (2005). On being able to be a couple: The importance of a "creative couple" in psychic life. In F. Grier (Ed.), *Oedipus and the couple* (pp. 9–30). London: Karnac.

Morgan, M. and Freedman, J. (2000). From fear of intimacy to perversion: A clinical analysis of the film *Sex, Lies and Videotape*. *British Journal of Psychotherapy*, 17(1): 85–93.

Ogden, T. H. (1989). On the concept of an autistic-contiguous position. *International Journal of Psycho-Analysis*, 70: 127–140.

O'Shaughnessy, E. (1964). The absent object. *Journal of Child Psychotherapy*, 1(2): 34–43.

Rosenthall, J. (2007). Sharing a heart: The dilemma of a fused couple. *British Journal of Psychotherapy*, 23(3): 411–429.

Royston, R. (2001). Sexuality and object relations. In C. Harding (Ed.), *Sexuality: psychoanalytic perspectives* (pp. 35–51). Hove: Brunner-Routledge.

Ruszczynski, S. (2020). Absent mindedness. *Unpublished paper presented at the 7th International Congress on Couple and Family Psychoanalysis*, San Francisco, 2020.

Waddell, M. (2002). *Inside lives: Psychoanalysis and the growth of the personality* (Revised Ed.). London: Karnac.

# Chapter 9

# Lesbian and gay couple relationships

## When internalised homophobia gets in the way of couple creativity

*Leezah Hertzmann*

Since the original publication of *"Lesbian and gay couple relationships: When internalised homophobia gets in the way of couple creativity"* over a decade ago (2011), many countries around the world have enshrined in law, rights for the LGBT community and those who face discrimination due to their sexual and gender identity. Simultaneously, there remain countries where persecution persists and where same-sex desire is a punishable criminal offence. However, progressive changes in the law which support the rights of individuals, and the greater acceptance of same-gender relationships, have not necessarily alleviated the internal conflicts for lesbian and gay couples of conscious and unconscious homophobia. The distress with which couples present in our consulting rooms still to this day, particularly that caused by the effects of internalised homophobia, warrants further consideration.

## Introduction

Many lesbian and gay couples remain cautious in seeking psychoanalytic treatment for their relationship difficulties. The use of psychoanalytic theories, particularly the application of the Oedipus complex to explore homosexuality has been experienced by many as especially damaging. It is regrettable that psychoanalytic theory has too often been used in a restrictive and deterministic way to pathologise sexual orientation. Yet, the concept of the Oedipus complex has also been immensely fruitful for psychoanalysis and remains one of its central tenets. In this paper I use the concept of the Creative Couple (Morgan, 2005), an idea which has evolved from the Oedipus complex, to underpin my thinking in an exploration of some of the

DOI: 10.4324/9781003265023-9

issues with which I have observed lesbian and gay couples strug-gle. One such issue is that of internalised homophobia. Using case examples, I consider the damage this can cause to lesbian and gay couples, including the sense of paralysis that can pervade both the couple's relationship and the therapy. I reflect on the challenges that internalised homophobia can present for the therapist when mani-fested in the transference and countertransference, and the need to be aware of the hidden, pernicious ways in which it can interfere with a couple's creativity.

Time and again, couples coming for therapy show us just how diffi-cult it can be to sustain an intimate adult couple relationship. According to psychoanalytic theories of couple relationships, partner choice involves conscious and unconscious aspects of the personality (Bannister et al., 1955). The strong bond a couple forms is understood to be a result of the union of their unconscious phantasies and pat-terns of relationships formed in early life. Each partner receives the other's unconscious projections giving a mutual feeling of acceptance and being understood. This mutual acceptance of the other's projec-tions constitutes an unconscious attachment that the couple will have to each other and will consist of shared internal phantasies and shared defences. These processes of projection and introjection form what has become known as the couple's projective system (Ruszczynski, 1993). In psychoanalytic couple psychotherapy, it is the couple's rela-tionship – their shared internal world, projective system, and interac-tional field which is the therapeutic focus and area of treatment, rather than either or both the individuals. When the couple's projective sys-tem is operating benignly, it can make those conflicted parts of the personality more tolerable and understood within oneself. However, when operating in a more destructive manner, it can also produce the effect of the need to control or attack this part of oneself which, now located in the other, can be more clearly seen.

Psychoanalytic couple psychotherapists are presented with the opportunity to observe and experience the ways couples demon-strate the significant aspects of their shared unconscious worlds in their relationship with each other, as well as with the therapist. In therapy, as couples begin to explain their difficulties, both the couple and the therapist become drawn into the emergent triangulated emo-tional experience. Each partner's fears, anxieties, conflicts as well as pleasures, phantasies, and hopes make up the couple's shared unconscious world and through the therapy, the rich internal life of the couple's relationship can become known.

## Application of psychoanalytic concepts to therapy with lesbian and gay couples

Lesbian and gay couples have been largely excluded from the rich body of psychoanalytic ideas and theories about couple relationships that has emerged over the last 60 years within the British psychoanalytic tradition (see Ruszczynski, 1993, for an overview). However, the North American psychoanalytic movement, with its shift away from drive theory in favour of a model more focused on relational and intersubjective techniques, has provided a fuller contribution to a largely relational psychoanalytic understanding of lesbian and gay couple relationships (for examples of this, see D'Ercole & Drescher, 2004; Domenici & Lesser, 1995).

One of the concepts from the British psychoanalytic tradition which I have used extensively in my work with couples – lesbian, gay, and heterosexual – is that of the "creative couple" (Morgan, 2005; Morgan & Ruszczynski, 1998). The creative couple is understood to be fundamentally a "state of mind" and is a belief in the need for and creativity of relationships. It is a recognition that we exist and function in the context of a relationship to another and it does not necessarily depend upon being in a relationship per se, as not every individual chooses to be part of a couple or achieves it if desired.

In applying the concept of the creative couple in therapeutic work with lesbian and gay couples, I have found that there can be a mirroring of the societal indictment of homosexuality reflected in the couple's relationship. This can interfere with the couple's capacity to inhabit a creative couple state of mind. In this paper, I want to consider how the homophobic discourse, potentially so pernicious, particularly when expressed by the couple themselves to attack each other and/or their relationship, may contribute to difficulties in sustaining the relationship. I draw on Britton's concept of the third position (Britton, 1989) and unconscious beliefs (Britton, 1998), as well as Kernberg's idea of the superego of the couple (Kernberg, 1995). Through case material, I will describe how I have used these psychoanalytic ideas to try to understand the particular expressions of the difficulties that occur for some lesbian and gay couples in their relationships.

## The creative couple state of mind and the relationship as a third

It is frequently the case that couples in difficulty find it hard to establish some objectivity about what is happening between them in their relationship. Morgan (2001) describes how symbolically the couple seeks this objectivity in the figure of the therapist. Here they hope to find a third that – *"can stand for the relationship, and this has a particular significance for the couple coming for help"* (Morgan, 2001, p. 19).

The therapist not only stands for the relationship, but simultaneously can stand outside it, while also inhabiting the relationship from the inside with the couple in the therapy. At the beginning, this capacity for objectivity rests with the therapist, but eventually it can become integrated in the couple themselves. An important part of this process of the therapy will be the coming together of the mind of the therapist with the minds of both partners in the couple. This can hopefully, in due course, enable them to be able to think about their relationship for themselves, generate a richer intercourse between them and establish a creative couple state of mind. The creative couple state of mind is, after all, an internal dialogue within ourselves from which our creative capacity comes and from which a rich internal life can develop and be shared with others.

The concept of the creative couple owes much to Britton's (1989) idea about a third position. This idea has its roots in Freud's discovery of the Oedipus complex, which he considered to be a central aspect of development (Freud, 1897, 1924) and later in what Klein named as the Oedipus Situation (Klein, 1928). Britton's idea about a third position is perhaps more closely related to Klein's conception of the Oedipus Situation – a triangular space within which a child experiences the following: the separate link with each parent, being the observer of and not participant in the parental couple relationship, and being observed by the parental couple. As Britton describes:

> If the link between the parents perceived in love and hate can be tolerated in the child's mind, it provides him with a prototype for an object relationship of a third kind in which he is a witness and not a participant. A third position then comes into existence from which object relationships can be observed. Given this, we can

also envisage being observed. This provides us with the capacity for seeing ourselves in interaction with others and for entertaining another point of view whilst retaining our own, for reflecting on ourselves while being observed.

(Britton, 1989, p. 87)

Gradually this capacity to observe oneself in one's own relationship becomes internalised as an aspect of oneself. The development of this third position is integral to the creative couple state of mind as there is an awareness of the relationship itself as a third, a new symbolic object. As the individuals create this new symbolic object between them and allow it to develop, there is a capacity for separateness and difference, an awareness of the fact of dependence and a capacity for self-reflection. In relative health, the relationship can then be subjectively experienced as a resource, an internal object in the relationship which both partners can turn to in their minds.

In couple relationships which function relatively well, when there is a disruption in the couple's relating to one another, each individual can take up the position of the relationship as a third, and observe him/herself within the relationship. The different or sometimes opposing perspective of one partner can be taken into the psyche of the other where it can be allowed to reside and join with one's own thoughts in a creative intercourse. This creativity becomes possible because a state of mind has been achieved in which two minds, and sometimes two bodies, can come together and create a third. Although for some couples this third may be the third of a child, for other couples it may be a different kind of third, more symbolic, something created together and nurtured, such as a shared endeavour.

The creative couple state of mind has then been discovered by the couple and can be recovered by them when things become difficult in their relationship. However, there may be many factors which interfere with the capacity to be a creative couple and maintain a creative couple state of mind. One such factor particularly pertinent to lesbian and gay couple relationships is the effect of internalised homophobia on couple functioning and I will now describe this further.

## Internalised homophobia – a perfect host for the couple's superego

Malyon (1982) described the struggle for internal acceptance of an individual's own sexuality and how this can, in part, lead to what he termed internalised homophobia. It is important to mention here that there has been a significant debate about the use of the term internalised homophobia and the concept it seeks to define which is beyond the scope of this paper (for further reading see Herek, 2004; Herek et al., 1998; Russell & Bohan, 2006). However, Malyon's definition of internalised homophobia, which emphasises shame, guilt, anger, hate, and disgust more than fear, is not entirely in accordance with psychoanalytic understanding and use of the term phobia. So, although internalised homophobia is not strictly speaking an analytic concept per se, I use it here because it is now widely referred to and generally understood to mean: *"the gay person's direction of negative social attitudes toward the self, leading to a devaluation of the self and resultant internal conflicts and poor self-regard ..."* (Meyer & Dean, 1998, p. 161).

In understanding the potentially destructive nature of internalised homophobia, it is necessary to think about the role of cultural and societal attitudes in relation to homosexuality, and how these impact and interact with the superego. Freud's development of the concept of the superego (1923) introduced the idea of a prohibitive and restrictive internal agent, a monument to parental authority and heir to the Oedipus complex. In "Civilization and its discontents" (1930), Freud put forward the idea of there being a strong link between the individual and the cultural superego. Both have origins in identifications with strong, authoritative figures who establish demands which make use of guilty feelings, particularly when these demands are not met. To link this with the concept of internalised homophobia, a person takes in ideas, judgements, and societal injunctions from the surrounding external world, alongside the widespread depictions of heterosexuality as the norm and homosexuality as abnormal or deviant. These elements become internalised and are then used directly to oppose, undermine, and attack his or her own sexual desires and sexual identity. Internalised homophobic content then becomes a component of the ego and functions both as an unconscious introject, as well as taking up a role in "influencing identity formation, self-esteem, the elaboration of defences, patterns of cognition, psychological integrity, and object relations" (Malyon, 1982). Therefore, what becomes internalised are object relationships that symbolically represent narratives expressing anti-homosexual attitudes and values (for further reading, see Downey & Friedman, 1995).

Over time the interaction of each partner's superego forges a new system which Kernberg (1993, 1995) calls the couple's superego. He describes how the couple relationship becomes the repository of both partners' conscious and unconscious phantasies, desires, and internalised object relations as well as conscious and unconscious superego functions. Kernberg stresses the importance of the benign function of the couple's superego, how the couple's mature superego -expressed in concern for the other as well as the self- protects the couple's object relations and fosters commitment and love. It contributes to a joint construction of values that serve as a boundary function for the couple in relation to the rest of the world. The couple can use these superego functions to creatively contribute to solving conflicts between them:

> ... an unexpected gesture of love, remorse, forgiveness, or humour may keep aggression within bounds. Tolerance of shortcomings and limitations in the other as well as in the self is silently integrated into the relationship.
>
> (Kernberg, 1995, p. 98)

The couple's superego also contains by its very nature remnants of Oedipal conflicts and therefore has the capacity for aggression, to threaten a couple's sexual love "by inhibiting or forbidding the expressions of tender and sexual feelings" (Kernberg, 1995, p. 97). Here Kernberg highlights how the couple's superego "may thus reinforce the capacity for lasting sexual passion or that very agency may destroy it" (1995, p. 97). For some lesbian and gay couples internalised homophobia can be an active component which may well influence whether the couple's superego reinforces or destroys aspects of their couple relationship.

I am suggesting here that internalised homophobia, functioning as an unconscious introject, acts as host for aggressive aspects of the superego potentially resulting in a very punitive attitude towards the homosexuality of the self and of others. In lesbian and gay couple relationships where internalised homophobia exists unconsciously in one or both partners, and therefore in their shared unconscious world, it can act as host for the couple's superego. Consequently, one's sexuality is repeatedly and persistently called into question not only by others, but inevitably by oneself. Crucially, it is not only that one's sexuality can feel scrutinised, different, or wrong, but in addition one's own sense of belief about oneself, and indeed about one's relationships, can come to feel equally under attack. This can have a particularly damaging effect on a couple's relationship and for some lesbian and gay couples, may contribute to difficulties in sustaining their relationship.

However, I would suggest that the introjection of internalised homophobia may also be considered a protective act aimed at adapting and transforming the unbearable pain of external attack into an apparently more stable, bearable position of internal indictment. Consequently, at an unconscious level there is a concordant view between external societal indictment and an internal indictment against homosexuality, which may play an important role in psychic stability. As a gay male patient recently said:

> Well at least if it's (internalised homophobia) inside me, then it is part of me. I don't have to worry so much about all that antigay stuff which is all around me because inside and outside all feel the same. I don't notice I attack myself then.

The difficulty with this is that such an adaptation may make the therapeutic endeavour even more challenging for therapists because of the profound human need for psychic stability and the couple's understandable reluctance to relinquish this. I have found that it is very important to try to investigate and grasp hold of the extent of a lesbian or gay couple's internalised homophobia in order to understand something of the landscape and size of the therapeutic task in hand. It may at first appear as though the couple is ego-syntonic in relation to their sexuality, but as the therapy progresses, it can become evident that the unconscious destructive aspects of internalised homophobia are operating within the couple relationship and that they are in fact ego-dystonic in relation to their sexuality. In my experience, internalised homophobia can be very resistant to the therapist's best efforts to address it. Just as it seems that some good therapeutic progress has been made, so it can be quickly undermined. A particularly persistent quality seems to emerge in the work where there is often a repetitious and immediate pull by the couple to use specific interactions as proof that their sexuality is wrong or abnormal, and also to attack both their sense of self and the relationship.

## Unconscious beliefs and internalised homophobia

Morgan (2010) describes how unconscious beliefs about being a couple and what a relationship is, form a central part of the unconscious life of the couple. She describes how unconscious beliefs have a particular feeling about them — although they are "beliefs" they reside in the unconscious like facts unless they become conscious and can be thought about. It is then that we become aware that they are in reality only beliefs. This idea shares much in common with Britton (1998), who described how something which starts as a belief can transform itself into an unconscious fact. These unconscious facts then become certainties which can drive many aspects of our conscious life. Britton gives a salient personal example of this, describing his own childhood belief in Father Christmas. It was only when he encountered another child who was more sceptical, that he realised –

*"Father Christmas was not a fact but a belief of mine."* The crucial point, which he puts so succinctly, is this:

> I needed the discovery that it was possible not to believe to discover that I had a belief and did not know a fact. It is the shift from thinking one knows a fact to realising one has a belief which is linked to self-awareness.
>
> (Britton, 1998, p. 14)

It is often the case that couples in difficulty present their thoughts and feelings about their partner as facts which the other – and frequently the therapist too – have to accept without question. It is possible to identify that this may be occurring when a couple's distress and arguments have a repetitive, fixed quality.

As the work of therapy progresses, it also becomes possible to see the way in which these unconscious facts drive much of what happens in the couple's relationship. Gradually, as a couple become aware of these unconscious facts, they can then shift from thinking they know a fact to realising that they have a belief. It is this capacity which can be so vital for the couple in developing insight into their relationship.

In my experience, lesbian and gay couples sometimes develop particular unconscious beliefs in relation to their sexuality. However, in the therapy it can take some time before these unconscious beliefs emerge because like many couples, lesbian and gay couples bring difficulties which need more immediate attention, consciously at least. Where internalised homophobia resides in the shared unconscious world of the couple and acts as host for the couple's superego, it can generate punitive unconscious beliefs along the lines of – "something about our coupling is bad, wrong, we shouldn't be like this or if only we weren't like this."

This can then prevent even the idea of a creative couple state of mind from fully emerging because something about the relationship itself is felt to be wrong. In the following composite example of therapy with a lesbian couple undertaken in a specialist unit for psychoanalytic couple psychotherapy, I want to illustrate how the very concept of their relationship came under attack from the effects of internalised homophobia. This lesbian couple was unable to use their relationship as an internal object to sustain and help them with their difficulties because their relationship itself was felt to be wrong. Just as the relationship could not be used as a resource, for a while, neither could the therapy.

*Clinical example*

Sasha and Rae had been in therapy for about 18 months. Over the past three months their relationship had been under a lot of stress due to the fact that Rae had been subject to a complaint at her workplace brought by a junior colleague to whom she thought she had been supportive. She was devastated that this had happened. Rae had been very distant and preoccupied with the complaint throughout this time and Sasha now felt worn out. The outcome of the internal investigation completely vindicated Rae, the employee left, and Rae was promoted. However, Rae remained preoccupied with the grievance and repeatedly played the details of the complaint in her mind. She described it as "a relentless record" in her head which she was powerless to switch off. It left her exhausted, ground down, and unable to enjoy anything including their sexual relationship together. They were unable to talk about what was happening in their relationship without it erupting into a huge argument with each insisting on their point, and they could not agree on even the simplest of things.

On one particular day, the couple arrived at their session looking very upset. Following another serious argument, they thought the only way forward was to separate. In the session they wondered if the grievance had precipitated some underlying difficulties which they believed were now impossible to address. The way in which they told the therapist about their impending separation and the reasons for it felt like an announcement. Unlike their previous way of relating to each other where they disagreed about most things, for the first time Rae and Sasha were aligned in their thinking and they both appeared to be utterly convinced of this shared belief about their relationship. The therapist's counter-transference was of being in a cul-de-sac and her attempts to help the couple think about their argument further were met with repeated rebuttals.

However, the therapist found her thoughts returning to the "relentless record" in Rae's mind. She wondered if her own attempts to engage the couple in thinking just now had perhaps been experienced by them as a relentless record. The therapist put this to the couple, who at first were irritated that she was returning to this seemingly unrelated issue now. The therapist none the less, without being really sure why, felt they should give this more thought and reluctantly they agreed.

This opened up an opportunity for Rae to describe the unremitting way in which her mind kept returning to the complaint, including the tormenting quality with which she attacked herself for the way she had managed her colleague. She said "*I know it's stupid, but I think if I were a better person, more patient and understanding, not a lesbian, bla bla bla, you* know… well, you know what I mean… then this wouldn't have happened." The therapist, aware of the patient's lack of coherence at this point, asked how being lesbian related to the grievance. Rae responded with something of a tirade:

Well, if you really want to know this is how it goes ... actually, it's like a rap or something in my mind. So, I'm bad because I'm lesbian, it's not the way it was supposed to be, gay relationships seldom last, probably because they're not normal anyway. It's like what my parents said when I came out to them – I do irreparable damage to others. That's what it's like.

A silence fell in the room, Rae became upset, and Sasha looked shocked. Eventually Sasha said that one of the things which had drawn her to Rae was that she seemed so comfortable with her sexuality, and this had helped Sasha herself to come out and to feel more at ease with her sexuality. Now this idea she had held about Rae was shattered and she felt that it had all been a sham. In this moment, it was as if there had been an unconscious agreement between Rae and Sasha which had now been severed.

I think it might be helpful to the reader to return to the idea of the couple's projective system mentioned previously (Ruszczynski, 1993) because it was in thinking about this that the therapist became able to see what might be happening between the couple. Sasha had found in Rae someone who was apparently at ease with her sexuality, as Sasha herself so wished to be. Simultaneously, Rae had found in Sasha someone who needed help to accept her sexuality and whom she could help to do so. In terms of partner choice, you could say there was a good unconscious fit between them. Rae could project her own introjected feelings of unconscious internalised homophobia into Sasha who, receiving this projection was then left holding the homophobic feelings for them both. In this way Rae could partly disown her unconscious feelings of internalised homophobia, while keeping this part of herself close by and locating it in Sasha, in whom there was already a valence. Then at a distance Rae could address these homophobic feelings in herself, but which were now located in Sasha. Now Rae was no longer unconsciously at risk of doing anyone "irreparable damage," in fact she was helping Sasha to grow and accept her sexuality. They had for some years maintained a stable and fulfilling relationship with their shared projective system working to support their couple relationship. However, the current accusation from her colleague seemed to have brought live in Rae a belief about herself as someone who would cause harm to others, which in her mind was linked to her parent's reaction when she came out. Symbolically the grievance had come to stand for Rae being guilty of causing "irreparable damage." Furthermore, it seemed that Sasha and Rae held a shared unconscious belief that lesbian and gay relationships never last. The therapist came up against their couple projective system which was in part being driven by their shared unconscious beliefs. What was striking about Rae and Sasha was that they had presented as ego-syntonic in relation to their sexuality and it was not until some apparently unrelated incident occurred, that their unconscious feelings about their sexuality could be known more consciously but in a very punitive way.

The therapist put something of her thoughts about the couple's projective system and their shared unconscious beliefs to them. She said that it felt as if they wanted her to be convinced just as they seemed to be, that there was something bad and deficient about them as a couple linked to being lesbian which was not amenable to change, and that this somehow meant their relationship had to end. There was a long silence and then Rae said *"For the first time it's like we are sitting on our own shoulders and watching what our private minds have been doing to our relationship."* Sasha said that she was shocked that they were just about to end their relationship and she added *"How on earth can we possibly look at our relationship more objectively if somewhere deep down inside, we think it's fundamentally wrong? There's no hope when it's like that."*

For Rae and Sasha, it was more difficult for both partners to use their relationship as an internal object and as a resource which they could turn to. The shared unconscious beliefs generated by internalised homophobia had interfered with their capacity for a creative couple state of mind. The therapist felt that it was important that she did not try to counter the couple's unconscious belief with another "fact," but instead explored the repetitive fixed quality of their belief to see where it led, and eventually something creative took place between all three. In putting things to the couple in a rather tentative way, the therapist's intention was to appeal to the more benign functions of the couple's superego which Kernberg describes (1993), rather than its more attacking and aggressive qualities. Eventually, Sasha and Rae could take in the therapist's thoughts alongside their own and allow something to develop out of this coming together. One might say a creative intercourse took place. The couple began to use both the therapy and their relationship as a resource they could turn to, their creative couple state of mind being more available to them now.

## Internalised homophobia and paralysis: the therapist as "homophobic other"

For many couples who come to therapy, part of their presenting problem and their complaint about their relationship will be that things feel stuck between them. With couples for whom this is the case, therapists frequently encounter a feeling of paralysis in their countertransference. In this respect Moss's (2002) work with individual gay men is equally useful in thinking about lesbian and gay couples. Moss describes how some gay men live out a conflicted relationship to their desired objects due to internalised homophobia in the following way: while simultaneously desiring the same-sex object, they also hit up against an internal repulsion and hatred of their own desire. According to Moss – "the founding opposition between desire and repulsion collapses, and the result is a fundamental stasis" (Moss, 2002, p. 7). For some lesbian and gay couples, this might mean that when they find a partner whom they desire and want to be in a couple relationship with, they inhabit a state of unconscious conflict and hatred in relation to their sexual object choice and also, I would say, towards their couple relationship. In the following example, I want to illustrate an earlier event with Sasha and Rae which occurred a few months into the therapy, where their shared internal sense of stasis had a paralysing effect both on their relationship and on the therapist. The way in which this paralysis became manifest was in a therapeutic injunction experienced by the therapist to not talk about the couple's sexuality and where the therapist then became the "homophobic other." In this way the couple could disavow themselves of their own feelings of internalised homophobia by projecting them into the therapist.

### Clinical example

Sasha and Rae had initially come for help as a couple because things had felt inexplicably stuck in their relationship for some time. They described how there was a constant push-pull dynamic between

them that had exerted an increasingly corrosive effect on their relationship and they were now very hostile and rejecting towards each
other. In the therapy, the therapist found that the couple constantly
rejected her interventions. At times she lost her train of thought and
wondered if there were aspects of the work that she was missing. In
looking at the work with her supervisor, together they noticed that
the therapist seemed to have bypassed a number of openings to talk
about their sexuality as it had emerged in the material. This surprised
the therapist given that she was experienced in working with lesbian
and gay couples and would not normally have sidestepped issues in
this way.

Subsequently, when further similar material was brought to the session by the couple, the therapist's attempts to explore the issues were
met with a defensive response and an accusation by the couple that
her curiosity indicated that she was homophobic. The therapist carefully considered this and became aware that in fact she felt she was
living with an injunction to not look at the couple's sexuality. Despite
feeling that it was important not to bypass the opportunity to help the
couple explore their feelings about their sexuality, in her countertransference she simultaneously felt paralysed. An opportunity presented
itself again, this time in relation to a party invitation at Sasha's workplace where staff usually brought partners and family. Sasha was not
out to colleagues at work and did not want Rae to come with her to
the party, and this had caused a nasty argument between them. When
the therapist asked about this, Sasha became very irritated and said –
*"Look, will you stop going on about this, ok?!… Just put a sock in it. I
don't want to think and I don't want to be lesbian. So that's that."* This
powerful statement said with such emotion momentarily left both the
couple and the therapist feeling taken aback. However, it provided a
pivotal moment in the therapy because it subsequently became possible for the couple to begin to explore their sexuality further. As the
work continued, this occasion was often referred to by the couple as
the moment where they began to know about the extent of their own
homophobic feelings and how these had become internalised within
their couple relationship.

For Sasha and Rae, I think there was perhaps a shared unconscious
belief in relation to their paralysis along the lines of – *"well if we keep
ourselves in this state of paralysis, we don't have to fully know about*

*or own our sexuality, which we would encounter through the other's response to our desire."* Ruth Stein (1998a, 1998b) lucidly describes how the pleasure of erotic desire comes from being able to transpose oneself in fantasy, into a state of mind which is felt to be the other's. For Sasha and Rae as a couple, their internal repulsion of their sexual desire for the other paralysed this ability. The wish not to know about or own their sexuality was manifested in the transference to the therapist who became the homophobic other. In her countertransference the therapist hit up against her own internal paralysis and appeared to drop the subject of their sexuality from her mind. She experienced an internal embargo, a therapeutic injunction, on thinking about the couple's sexuality and her attempts to do so were seen by the couple as her homophobia.

The stasis in the couple's relationship which paralysed the therapist's mind made it difficult for the therapist to find a third position from which to observe what was occurring in the therapy. This was eventually found in the supervisor who was able to help the therapist observe what was happening in the work. At this moment one might say that the therapist and supervisor were able to inhabit something of a creative couple state of mind in relation to the therapy with Sasha and Rae. Morgan (2005) emphasises the importance of the belief in relationships as a source of creativity not just through concretely becoming part of a couple, but also through contact with colleagues, friends, and even good internal objects. Just as therapists consult with colleagues who are particularly experienced in working with specific patient populations, this may also be necessary when clinicians are working with lesbian and gay couples. Certainly, in the case of Sasha and Rae, it helped the therapy to take a more productive turn.

## Concluding thoughts

In this paper, I have drawn attention to the pernicious and damaging effects of internalised homophobia on lesbian and gay couple relationships and the accompanying challenges for therapists, particularly a sense of paralysis, therapeutic injunctions, and the therapist as homophobic other. Internalised homophobia is just one of the issues that can jeopardise sustaining a satisfying, creative couple relationship.

The psychoanalytic ideas used in this paper have helped me to explore some of the therapeutic challenges attendant in working with this powerful and sometimes hidden force.

Inevitably, space has precluded the exploration of other important issues relevant to this subject, particularly those of the therapist's own sexual orientation and issues of analytic neutrality. However, I do want to briefly consider something of the biological aspects of lesbian and gay relationships which can potentially present further conflicts. In my experience, there can be a real need for lesbian and gay couples to mourn the fact that they cannot biologically create another life through their intercourse and have a baby with their part- ner in this way. Many lesbian and gay couples do indeed have children and achieve this in a variety of ways, finding different and creative family formations in which to raise their children. Even when a cou- ple have already become parents together by other means, for some there is an intense feeling of resentment that their partner is not able to give them a baby. To address this issue, particularly when it is unconscious, can be delicate and painful work in therapy. For a het- erosexual couple their sexual life and the act of their intercourse together can result in the creativity of another life. The opportunities that now exist for lesbian and gay couples to have children could divert attention away from the conflicts that may exist as a result of the biological impossibility of creating a baby together. Sandler (2006) describes how in making this point some would call her hom- ophobic for doing so and yet, not to fully consider the impact of this reality would be to overlook the centrality in psychoanalysis of Freud's theory of development where the body, sexuality and desire are intrinsic to mental life (Freud, 1905, 1924). In my opinion, not considering this biological aspect is to leave something crucial unexplored.

In the process of writing this paper and returning to psychoanalytic theories of sexuality, it is noticeable how some concepts have been misused in a homophobic and moralistic way. Milton (2000) warns more generally of the way in which derailments of a psychoanalytic standpoint can easily occur, where the moral high ground is then assumed, and theories become "morally loaded concepts."

What is clear now though is that within psychoanalysis a more exploratory, less judgemental zeitgeist is emerging with regard to sexuality. For instance, Target (2007) and Fonagy (2008) have both in different ways put forward ideas that seek to re-centre psychosexuality at the heart of analytic enquiry and redress the previous theoretical pull in the direction of understanding psychosexuality mostly as an expression of early object relationships. Put briefly, both authors describe the central importance that mirroring of affect by the primary caregiver plays in the capacity for emotional regulation. However, the uniqueness of sexual experience means that caregivers repeatedly leave unmirrored expressions of infantile sexuality, which in turn means that sexual feelings remain dysregulated in us all. These ideas and those described in other recent publications (Fonagy et al., 2006; Stein, 1998a, 1998b) illustrate a move to place psychosexuality and the biological aspects of psychoanalysis more centrally. This opens up possibilities for a fuller understanding of how our sexual identity and gender come to be authentically felt in each of us.

Finally, it is probably true to say that we can help our patients only in as much as we have worked on our own feelings about our sexuality, gender, and our own internalised homophobia, regardless of our sexual orientation. We are less likely to be able to understand these aspects in our patients if we do not understand them within ourselves. This is always work in progress and by its very nature, not something ever completed and arrived at.

## References

Bannister, K., Lyons, A., Pincus, L., Robb, J., Shooter, A., & Stephens, J. (1955). *Social casework in marital problems*. London: Tavistock Publications.

Britton, R. (1989). The missing link: Parental sexuality in the Oedipus complex. In J. Steiner (Ed.), *The Oedipus complex today: Clinical implications* (pp. 83–101). London: Karnac Books.

Britton, R. (1998). *Belief and imagination: Explorations in psychoanalysis*. London: Routledge.

D'Ercole, A., & Drescher, J. (2004). *Uncoupling convention: Psychoanalytic approaches to same-sex couples and families*. Hillsdale, NJ: The Analytic Press.

Domenici, T., & Lesser, R.C. (1995). *Disorienting sexuality: Psychoanalytic reappraisals of sexual identities*. New York: Routledge.

Downey, J.I., & Friedman, R.C. (1995). Internalized homophobia in lesbian relationships. *Journal of the American Academy of Psychoanalysis*, 23, 435–447.

Fonagy, P. (2008). A genuinely developmental theory of sexual enjoyment and its implications for psychoanalytic technique. *Journal of the American Psychoanalytic Association*, 56(1), 11–36.

Fonagy, P., Krause, R., & Leuzinger-Bohleber, M. (2006). *Identity, gender and sexuality: 150 years after Freud.* London: Karnac Books.

Freud, S. (1897). Letter 71. Extracts from the Fliess papers. Standard Edition, 1.

Freud, S. (1905). Three essays on the theory of sexuality. Standard Edition, 7.

Freud, S. (1923). The ego and the id. Standard Edition, 19.

Freud, S. (1924). The dissolution of the Oedipus complex. Standard Edition, 19.

Freud, S. (1930). Civilization and its discontents. Standard Edition, 21.

Herek, G.M. (2004). Beyond "homophobia": Thinking about sexual prejudice and stigma in the twenty-first century. *Sexuality Research and Social Policy*, 1, 6–24.

Herek, G.M., Cogan, J.C., Gillis, J.P., & Glunt, E.K. (1998). Correlates of internalized homophobia in a community sample of lesbians and gay men. *Journal of the Gay and Lesbian Medical Association*, 2, 17–25.

Kernberg, O.F. (1993). The couple's constructive and destructive superego functions. *Journal of the American Psychoanalytic Association*, 41(3), 653–677.

Kernberg, O.F. (1995). Superego functions. In O. Kernberg (Ed.), *Love relations: Normality and pathology* (pp. 97–112). New Haven, CT: Yale University Press.

Klein, M. (1928). Early stages of the Oedipus conflict. *International Journal of Pyscho-Analysis*, 9, 167–180 (reprinted in Love, guilt and reparation. London: Hogarth Press, 1975).

Malyon, A.K. (1982). Psychotherapeutic implications of internalized homophobia in gay men. *Journal of Homosexuality*, 7, 59–69.

Meyer, I.H., & Dean, L. (1998). Internalized homophobia, intimacy, and sexual behaviour among gay and bisexual men. In G.M. Herek (Ed.), *Stigma and sexual orientation: Understanding prejudice against lesbians, gay men and bisexuals* (pp. 160–186). Thousand Oaks, CA: Sage.

Milton, J. (2000). Psychoanalysis and the moral high ground. *International Journal of Psycho-Analysis*, 81(6), 1101–1116.

Morgan, M. (2001). First contacts: The therapist's "couple state of mind" as a factor in the containment of couples seen for consultation. In F. Grier (Ed.), *Brief encounters with couples* (pp. 17–32). London: Karnac Books.

Morgan, M. (2005). On being able to be a couple: The importance of a "creative couple" in psychic life. In F. Grier (Ed.), *Oedipus and the couple* (pp. 9–30). London: Karnac Books.

Morgan, M. (2010). Unconscious beliefs about being a couple. *Fort Da*, 16A(1):36–55.

Morgan, M., & Ruszczynski, S. (1998). The creative couple. Unpublished paper presented at the Tavistock Marital Studies Institute 50th Anniversary Conference.

Moss, D. (2002). Internalized homophobia in men: Wanting in the first person singular, hating in the first person plural. *Psychoanalytic Quarterly*, 71(1), 21–50.

Russell, G.M., & Bohan, J.S. (2006). The case of internalized homophobia: Theory and/as practice. *Theory and Psychology*, 16, 343–366.

Ruszczynski, S. (1993, reprinted in 2005). *Psychotherapy with couples: Theory and practice at the Tavistock Institute of Marital Studies.* London: Karnac Books.

Sandler, A.-M. (2006). Commentary on "The issues of homosexuality in psychoanalysis" by R.C. Friedman. In P. Fonagy, R. Krause, & M. Leuzinger-Bohleber (Eds) *Identity, gender and sexuality: 150 years after Freud* (pp. 98–102). London: Karnac.

Stein, R. (1998a). The enigmatic dimension of sexual experience: The "otherness" of sexuality and primal seduction. *Psychoanalytic Quarterly*, 67, 594–625.

Stein, R. (1998b). The poignant, the excessive and the enigmatic in sexuality. *International Journal of Psycho-Analysis*, 79, 253–268.

Target, M. (2007). Is our sexuality our own? A developmental model of sexuality based on early affect mirroring. *British Journal of Psychotherapy*, 23(4), 517–530.

# Chapter 10

# Discussion of "Lesbian and gay couple relationships"

## When internalised homophobia gets in the way of couple creativity

*Gary Grossman*

There is now a wealth of literature addressing a range of perspectives on psychoanalytic couple therapy with heterosexual couples. However, as Leezah Hertzmann pointedly notes in her chapter, there continues to be few psychoanalytic contributions to therapy with lesbian and gay couples. In addition to drawing attention to the unique experiences of lesbians and gay men that impact a couple's relationship, I read Hertzman's chapter as also demonstrating how psychoanalytic models of couples have neglected the role of the socio-cultural in theorising the construction of intimate relationships.

Hertzmann specifically draws on the concept of the "creative couple" (Morgan, 2005, 2020), an internally constructed capacity and "state of mind," that forms via psychological development. She recognises the impact of culture on the psychological development and internal world of each member of a same-sex couple by honing in on internalised homophobia and its potential to "… interfere with the couple's capacity to inhabit a creative couple state of mind" (this volume, p. 114). Internalised homophobia, though not a strictly psychoanalytic concept (as Hertzmann notes), provides a framework for recognising the processes by which a lesbian or gay man has unconsciously absorbed society's denigration of homosexuality and idealisation of heterosexuality over the course of early psychic development. Consequently, when the child first encounters conscious same-sex erotic fantasies and desires, it is within an internal world that prohibits and maligns such desires. Through her clinical vignette, Hertzmann illustrates how internalised homophobia can interfere in the formation of a creative couple state of mind.

Homophobia refers to hostility and/or antipathy towards and bias and/or prejudice against homosexuals, homosexual behaviour, or culture. Homophobia has become a common, catchall term to describe

DOI: 10.4324/9781003265023-10

negative attitudes towards homosexuals and homosexuality (Auchincloss & Samberg, 2012). Homophobia is a cross-cultural phenomenon. Heterosexuality is privileged in every society and although progress towards equity has advanced in some parts of the world, there are still no cultures that value and celebrate same-sex sexuality and relationships on equal footing with other-sex sexuality and relationships. Every adult who identifies as lesbian, gay, bi or queer has both absorbed these cultural attitudes towards their sexuality and has journeyed through a process of reconciling their erotic desires and identity with society's prejudices. "Internalised homophobia" has become the common usage for describing the incorporation of society's anti-homosexual bias within the internal world of a gay man or lesbian.

Understanding the psychological processes that lead to the internalisation of societal homophobia is essential in understanding its impact on the intimate relationships of lesbians and gay men. Hertzmann conceptualises the internalisation of homophobia as a component of superego development. Within Freud's structural theory, the superego is one of the three components of the personality, along with id and ego, and is established via identifications with parental objects through the resolution of the Oedipus Complex. It is through this process that the child internalises their culture's mores and values. The superego establishes an "ego ideal," based on the child's culture and transmitted by their parent/s, by which the self is measured and either praised or criticised. Parents transmit their fantasies of who their child is and will become. With heterosexuality as a universal norm, parents are most likely to imagine their child falling in love with a member of the other sex and conforming to gender-typical interests and behaviours. Hertzmann elaborates her theory of superego formation and internalised homophobia by drawing more explicitly on an Object Relations theory of development: "… what becomes internalised are object relationships that symbolically represent narratives expressing anti-homosexual attitudes and values …" (this volume, p. 118). A further elaboration of the processes involved in the internalisation of homophobia will, I believe, enhance a therapist's capacity to recognise the impact of internalised homophobia when their lesbian and gay couples are not aware of it.

In a subsequent paper, Hertzmann (2015) provides a more detailed account of the child's developing internal object relational world through the lens of emerging sexuality. Drawing on the studies of

Target (2007) and Fonagy (2008) on disruptions of parental mirroring of infant sexual excitement, Hertzmann suggests that the unmarked and unelaborated response may have a more adverse impact on psychosexual development for the child who later identifies as lesbian or gay. Within a heterocentric society, parents are likely more able to recognise and tolerate sexual excitement in a child of the other sex than with a child of the same sex.

> ... where the parental response to a child's expression of same-gender desire and emerging sexuality in childhood is unwelcoming, then the trajectory and eventual fate of identifications with both parents, as well as the capacity to experience and inhabit one's innate bisexuality, will be significantly affected ... where a child's emergent sexual orientation is different to that of their parents, the parents' responses to sexual arousal in a child of the same-gender as themselves may be to react with an even greater degree of alarm, disapproval, or disgust which in turn the child then internalizes.
>
> (Hertzmann, 2015, p. 160)

Beginning with Isay's (1987, 1989) reconceptualisation of the Oedipal phase for boys who grow up to identify as gay, numerous analytic writers have revitalised a multifaceted and varied understanding of the Oedipal experience and its impact on development in lesbians and gay men freed from heterocentric bias (Davies, 2015; Elise, 2002; Goldsmith, 1995, 2001; Nathans, 2021; Phillips, 2001; Rose, 2007). Nathans (2021) chooses the Kleinian "Oedipal Situation" over the traditional "Oedipus Complex" as a more inclusive, varied, and flexible framework for understanding triadic development unmoored from heterosexual assumption. In all of these models, the Oedipal Situation involves the unconscious world of child and parents, incorporating the parents' fantasies about their child and responses to their child's erotic attachments and pursuits.

In her 2015 paper, Hertzmann considers the unique Oedipal Situation for lesbians and gay men as a lens for understanding the impact of the internal parental couple on their adult couple relationships. The incongruity between the erotic life of lesbians or gay men and that of their heterosexual parents may lead to a rejection of the internal parental couple, potentially leading to challenges in adult intimate partnerships. Hertzmann's 2015 paper is essential, I believe, in bringing greater appreciation to the impact of internalised homophobia on lesbian and gay couples that she describes in this volume.

In her exploration of internalised homophobia within lesbian and gay couples, Hertzmann highlights the tenacity of attacks against the self and its potential to impede therapy. She understands the persistence of this internal indictment of sexuality as a protective measure: by transforming an external attack into an internal attack, the individual creates a sense of mastery over the injury. Although a couple may appear to be comfortable and accepting of their sexuality and their queer identities, unconscious homophobia emerges as the therapy progresses. "In my experience, internalised homophobia can be very resistant to the therapist's best efforts to address it" (this volume, p. 119). Recognising internalised homophobia's roots in early Oedipal empathic failures and rejection further accounts for the tenacity of these anti-gay attitudes and beliefs.

Oedipal rejections and empathic failures can lead to the development of internal self-representations as faulty, lacking, repellent, dangerous and, therefore, unlovable and object representations as critical, disapproving, disgusted, frightened, and rejecting. The array of anti-gay attitudes a lesbian or gay adolescent is confronted with will resonate with their pre-existing unconscious internal self-object world. As a result, the adolescent is especially vulnerable to rejections related to their emerging sexuality, increasing the likelihood of identification with the aggressor as a means of defence. As the teen internalises these anti-gay attitudes, they reinforce their pre-existing, Oedipally derived unconscious beliefs about themself and their objects.

It has been my experience with many of the gay and lesbian patients I have treated that, in contrast to overt attitudes towards homosexuality, underlying anti-gay convictions are resilient and persistent throughout adulthood, and are resistant to modification through ordinary experience. For a lesbian or gay man, early experiences of hostility and rejection towards their homosexuality are conscious or pre-conscious and capable of being remembered and, therefore, reflected upon and revised. In contrast, Oedipal experiences of rejection, hostility, and humiliation are repressed and, without intervention, remain unconscious. And because these experiences are unconscious, they are shielded and remain in their original form, unmodified by experience or through emotional and intellectual maturity. As adolescent and adult lesbian and gay men negotiate coming out, they have the opportunity to confront and modify their conscious homophobia, and often feel a sense of resolution and acceptance of being lesbian or gay. Underlying anti-gay attitudes, linked with the denied romance of their Oedipal years, however, persist in their unaltered form. It is this unconscious link between Oedipal rejection, along with the formation of associated internal self and object representations, and the identification with society's aggression towards homosexuality, that accounts for the persistence of internalised homophobia in openly gay and lesbian individuals.

Hertzmann draws our attention to the role of unconscious beliefs in the formation of a couple. Until an unconscious belief becomes accessible to awareness and self-reflection, it continues to inform an individual's experiences of themselves and in relationship, as if a fact. An unconscious belief can likely be formed at any point across the lifespan. However, our earliest beliefs, formed and repressed prior to emotional and intellectual maturity and during the period of infantile narcissism, are especially likely to be distorted and ego-centric, such as the beliefs derived from the child's Oedipal experiences of rejection and empathic failure. The child whose erotic longings are ignored, rejected, or derided may readily develop the belief that there is something wrong with, or bad about, them. As Hertzmann points out, this easily transforms in adult intimate relationships to the belief that there is something wrong with us as a couple.

Hertzmann provides us with an evocative clinical illustration of various expressions and the impact of internalised homophobia in a lesbian couple. We might consider Sasha and Rae to be a discordant couple, with Rae apparently more comfortable about her sexuality and openly lesbian throughout her life, and Sasha less accepting of her sexuality and openly lesbian in parts of her life, but closeted at work. Sasha's internalised homophobia is more conscious and accessible, as revealed early in the therapy during an angry reaction to their therapist's curiosity about excluding Rae from a work party, "Look, will you stop going on about this, ok?! … Just put a sock in it. I don't want to think and I don't want to be lesbian …" (this volume, p. 126). This became a pivotal moment in the couple therapy, as Hertzmann describes, "… this occasion was often referred to by the couple as the moment where they began to know about the extent of their own homophobic feelings and how these had become internalized within their couple relationship" (this volume, p. 127). Although it appears as though the couple could then begin to address the homophobia in their relationship, later in the treatment it became evident that Sasha was carrying the homophobic feelings and beliefs for both of them. Rae, who had appeared as accepting and at ease with her sexuality, revealed her own struggles with being a lesbian in the context of a work conflict. As Rae exposed her beliefs that it is bad to be lesbian and that gay relationships are wrong and abnormal, the therapist was better able to see, and help her patients see, the projective systems at play that drew and held this couple together. As the couple's shared unconscious beliefs about their sexuality became accessible, the couple was able to retreat from their sudden intent to separate, and were able to reflect on the impact of internalised homophobia on their relationship.

Hertzmann addresses the various ways that unconscious homophobic beliefs may be managed within a couple therapy, recognising the function of disavowal and projection within the couple and between the couple and the therapist. Not infrequently, this results in the anti-gay beliefs being located in the therapist. In order to effectively process and work with these transference projections, Hertzmann advises that the therapist must make the effort to discover, reflect on, and interrogate their own unconscious biases towards homosexuality.

In addition to contributing to the development of internalised homophobia in lesbians and gay men, the socio-cultural surround also plays a prominent role in the individual's capacity to recognise continuing internal anti-gay attitudes and beliefs. As a gay psychoanalyst practising in San Francisco for over 40 years, I have rarely seen an adult patient, as an individual or part of a couple, who expressed or was aware of negative attitudes or beliefs about their sexuality early in the treatment. The majority of these patients moved to San Francisco after coming out and, for many, the reputation of the "City by the Bay" as a safe haven for gay men and lesbians was a determining draw. Most had become involved in the local lesbian, gay, bisexual, and transgender (LGBT) community, through the bar/nightclub scene, LGBT rights and cultural organisations, and AIDS/HIV activism, and established a social network of other lesbians and gay men. For these gay men and lesbians, earlier struggles with accepting their sexuality had been consciously and intentionally worked through and seemingly resolved, and they found reinforcement, affirmation, and support for this acceptance from their community. This has been especially true in the gay male couples I have worked with. Although there are certainly exceptions, in my experience as a therapist, coupled gay men in San Francisco are more likely to be publicly out, consider themselves to be accepting of and comfortable with their sexuality, and do not consider the possibility that internalised homophobia contributes to the challenges that prompted them to seek therapy. In both individual and couple therapy, it is often the therapist who recognises the underlying anti-gay beliefs and then must help the patient or couple uncover their internalised homophobia. For example, unconscious attitudes and beliefs about homosexuality may be reflected in self-destructive behaviours such as substance abuse and reckless or risky sexual behaviour, or pervasive feelings of worthlessness, or loss of sexual interest in their partner. In gay men, internalised homophobia is often linked to unconscious identifications with society's devaluing of women and femininity. As a sequela of the proto-gay boy's erotic longing for his father, he may be especially motivated to identify with his mother in his efforts to win his father's attention, linking his homo-eroticism with feminine identifications, and this may account for the divergence from traditional male gender roles in many gay boys and men. Interest in bodybuilding and the pursuit of a hard-muscled physique, widely endorsed and valued in gay male culture, may serve to defend against these early feminine identifications and reflect unconscious attacks on his same-sex desires.

Another framework where internalised homophobia may shed light on a lesbian or gay couple's sexual dissatisfaction involves the role of aggression in erotic excitement and pleasure (Kernberg, 1991). If we understand the formation of internalised homophobia as the dynamic outcome of the child's defensive response to environmental hostility and rejection of their sexuality, we can see a complicated link with aggression. By turning passive into active, the child identifies with the aggressor, effectively warding off vulnerability, injury, and humiliation, while internalising the hostility and derision of their sexuality. In the experience of coming out and working through conscious negative attitudes and beliefs about their homosexuality and developing a positive lesbian or gay identity, the lesbian or gay man may also need to disavow their aggressive strivings in the process of relinquishing their hostility and rejection of same-sex desires. This may account for the presenting complaints in therapy of "lesbian bed death" (Iasenza, 2002; van Rosmalen-Nooijens et al., 2008) in long-term female couples and sexual incompatibility reported by gay male couples.

As Western societies have become increasingly accepting, acknowledging, and valuing of same-sex relationships, children who grow up and identify as bisexual, lesbian, or gay have experienced greater possibilities for developing positive images of themselves and their sexuality. Concurrently with this progress, there continue to be communities in which homosexuality is explicitly condemned, families that have trouble accepting their LGBT children, and political and social forces that privilege heterosexual relationships over same-sex relationships. As a result, the absorption of anti-gay attitudes and beliefs is a persistent emotional challenge for gay men and lesbians, individually and within their romantic partnerships.

Hertzmann's contributions to our psychoanalytic understanding of lesbian and gay couples in therapy have provided a necessary appreciation of the socio-cultural surround. Her attention to the presence of internalised homophobia, especially when outside of the couples' awareness, reminds us of its potential to disrupt relationship satisfaction. Hertzmann's clinical vignette provides an example of a couple with one member who is aware of her negative attitudes towards her lesbianism, and the other who becomes aware of her biases only through the course of therapy. Therapists, I believe, are presented with unique challenges and opportunities when both members of a lesbian or gay couple present as accepting and comfortable with their sexuality, with no conscious awareness of anti-gay attitudes or beliefs. Understanding the early developmental underpinnings of internalised homophobia, linked to Oedipal rejection and empathic failure, and common expressions of unconscious anti-gay beliefs, will better prepare therapists to recognise its impact on their lesbian and gay couples.

## References

Auchincloss, E.L. & Samberg, E. (2012). *Psychoanalytic terms and concepts.* New Haven: Yale University Press.

Davies, J.M. (2015). From Oedipus Complex to Oedipal complexity: Reconfiguring (pardon the expression) the negative Oedipal Complex and the disowned erotics of disowned sexualities. *Psychoanalytic Dialogues, 25,* 265–283.

Elise, D. (2002). The primary maternal Oedipal Situation and female homoerotic desire. *Psychoanalytic Inquiry, 22*(2), 209–258.

Fonagy, P. (2008). A genuinely developmental theory of sexual enjoyment and its implications for psychoanalytic technique. *Journal of the American Psychoanalytic Association, 56*(1), 11–36.

Goldsmith, S.J. (1995). Oedipus or Orestes? Aspects of gender identity development in homosexual men. *Psychoanalytic Inquiry*, *15*, 112–124.

Goldsmith, S.J. (2001). Oedipus or Orestes? Homosexual men, their mothers, and other women revisited. *Journal of the American Psychoanalytic Association*, *49*, 1269–1287.

Hertzmann, L. (2015). Objecting to the object: Encountering the internal parental couple relationship for lesbian and gay couples. In A. Lemma & P. Lynch *Sexualities: Contemporary psychoanalytic perspectives* (pp. 156–174). London & New York: Routledge.

Iasenza, S. (2002) Beyond "Lesbian bed death": The passion and play in lesbian relationships. *Journal of Lesbian Studies*, *6*(1), 111–120.

Isay, R. (1987). Fathers and their homosexually inclined sons in childhood. *Psychoanalytic Study of the Child*, *42*, 275–294.

Isay, R. (1989). *Being homosexual: Gay men and their development*. New York: Farrar, Straus, & Giroux.

Kernberg, O. (1991). Aggression and love in the relationship of the couple. *Journal of the American Psychoanalytic Association*, *39*, 45–70.

Morgan, M. (2005). On being able to be a couple: The importance of a "creative couple" in psychic life. In F. Grier (Ed.), *Oedipus and the couple* (pp. 191–205). London: Karnac Books.

Morgan, M. (2020). Being a couple and developing the capacity for creative parenting: A psychoanalytic perspective. *Journal of Child Psychotherapy*, *46*(2), 191–205.

Nathans, S. (2021). Oedipus for everyone: Revitalizing the model for LGBTQ couples and single parent families. *Psychoanalytic Dialogues*, *31*(3), 312–328.

Phillips, S. (2001). The overstimulation of everyday life: I. New aspects of male homosexuality. *Journal of the American Psychoanalytic Association*, *49*(4), 1235–1268.

Rose, S. (2007). *Oedipal rejection: Echoes in the relationships of gay men*. Youngstown, NY: Cambria Press.

Target, M. (2007). Is our sexuality our own? A developmental model of sexuality based on early affect mirroring. *British Journal of Psychotherapy*, *23*(4), 517–530.

van Rosmalen-Nooijens, K., Vergeer, C., & Lagro-Janssen, A. (2008) Bed death and other lesbian sexual problems unraveled: A qualitative study of the sexual health of lesbian women involved in a relationship. *Women & Health*, *48*(3), 339–362.

# Chapter 11

# Lost – and found – in translation

## Do Ronald Fairbairn's ideas still speak usefully to 21st-century couple therapists?

*Molly Ludlam*

### Introduction

This chapter aims to consider whether Ronald Fairbairn's ideas can be said to have made a lasting contribution to current Object Relations couple psychotherapy. In some circles, Fairbairn is known as the father, and Melanie Klein as the mother, of Object Relations therapy. Interestingly, however, in these days of single parenting, with mothers, in particular, going it alone, Klein is often identified as if she is the singlehanded mother of "Object Relations," while Fairbairn's role as father, especially in Kleinian circles, is completely forgotten or ignored. The desire to honour Fairbairn explains, in part, some of the reasoning behind my choice of title, "Lost – and found – in translation." I also want to emphasise the difficulties there have been in understanding Fairbairn's language, alongside the "translation" and recognition of his ideas, that have enabled them to be used as a secure base from which to develop psychoanalytic thinking. My particular focus, however, is on the fundamental role his concepts have played in developing couple psychoanalytic psychotherapy.

The difficulties Fairbairn's work has encountered in being taken in and acknowledged raise questions about what it is that gets in the way when we try to convey our thoughts. Native English speakers in Britain and the US are often said to be divided by a common language, making the potential for misunderstanding ever present. In the UK, there is a saying: "What counts is not what you say, but the way that you say it." Psychotherapists know, of course, that *both* matter. *What* you say and *how* you say it affect not only how you are understood, but whether you are taken seriously. Certainly, this was Fairbairn's experience. Like many other psychoanalytic thinkers, he created his own language, but in doing so, he struggled to find terms that his peers would readily

DOI: 10.4324/9781003265023-11

adopt as useful and authoritative. As a result, many of the ideas of this unassuming Scot did get "lost" in the London-centred, psychoanalytic world of his day.

Fairbairn, like all great psychoanalytic theorists, was both visionary in his thinking and limited by his own experience. A brief introduction to the man and his time will serve to place him in context.

## Brief biography

An only child, Ronald Fairbairn was born in 1889 into a well-to-do, and strictly Calvinist, Edinburgh family. He was well-educated; his first degree at Edinburgh University in "Mental Philosophy" gave him a good grounding in the Classics, and Aristotelian and Hegelian philosophy. His first ambition was to go into the Church, but he was diverted into military service by the First World War. During that time, he was very impressed by visiting William Rivers, who was treating shell-shocked patients at Craiglockhart War Hospital in Edinburgh. Pat Barker's trilogy, *Regeneration* (Barker, 1996) recounts Rivers' work. When the war ended, Fairbairn felt he could best help others as a psychoanalyst. After two periods of analysis in London and Edinburgh, he trained as a medical doctor, specialising in psychiatry. He considered completing his training at the Tavistock Clinic in London, but, being now married and with a family, he decided to stay in Edinburgh, where he developed a private psychotherapy practice. His university teaching post in psychology also involved him in clinical work with adults, and with children at a Child Guidance Clinic.

Fairbairn was an avid reader of psychoanalytic literature, reading Freud in German, as well as in translation, and thanks to the links he had cultivated with London colleagues, in 1931, he presented a clinical paper to the British Psycho-Analytical Society and was elected an Associate member (Fairbairn, 1931). That meant he was eligible to attend its London meetings, so that he became familiar with Melanie Klein's work, and she with his. For example, Fairbairn introduced the idea of the schizoid position to Klein. Their mutual respect and awareness probably helped each of them to develop their own distinctive voice. Practising in Edinburgh, 400 miles north of London, risked being a lonely and professionally isolating experience for Fairbairn, although it may have fitted well with his independent-mindedness. Being an outsider fostered a freedom to question orthodoxies. It also helped Fairbairn keep his distance from the acrimony of the Controversial Discussions of 1942–1944 between Melanie Klein and her followers and Anna Freud and her supporters. He found all that conflict, and the consequent rift in the British Psycho-Analytical Society, distasteful and unnecessary. Reflecting on this, we should not be surprised that, in the context of the war, splitting, and an interest in splitting, came into the heart of a society of practitioners dedicated to understanding the conflicts and tensions that afflicted their patients.

A middle group, later called the Independents, emerged in the mid-1940s. Although its members might have had much in common with the approach of both the Kleinian and Anna Freudian camps, the Independents preferred not to be allied with either of the adversaries. Along with Donald Winnicott, John Bowlby, Michael Balint, and others, Fairbairn came to be considered an Independent, and one who profoundly influenced that group's thinking. Indeed, the early 1940s proved a particularly creative time for him when he wrote four of his most important papers. They were later included in the 1952 major collection of his work *Psychoanalytic Studies of the Personality* (Fairbairn, 1952). Although he did not see himself as challenging Freud, this book significantly reframes psychoanalytic theory: "drive theory" and the "death instinct" are jettisoned and replaced by Fairbairn's own carefully constructed theory of internal Object Relations. Setting forth into new psychoanalytic territory, however, Fairbairn coined terms not previously used by other theorists: for example, "endopsychic structure," "central ego," "exciting object," "libidinal ego," "rejecting object," and "internal saboteur." His adoption of a new language unfortunately created barriers rather than bridges to understanding his creative, new theories. Consequently, his particular vocabulary has not found a place in common psychoanalytic discourse.

There are probably many explanations for any relative unfamiliarity with Fairbairn's theories compared with those of Klein. But how should we account for the fact that Winnicott, a fellow Independent, largely ignored him, despite the similarity in their approaches? Perhaps Fairbairn's implicit criticism of Freud made Winnicott and his contemporaries, after the recent bitter quarrelling, anxious about the risk of ostracism. While Heinz Kohut also clearly followed in Fairbairn's footsteps, curiously, he never cites him. We might wonder then whether Fairbairn's ideas were perhaps absorbed into the zeitgeist and reproduced without being attributed. Certainly, he was writing at a time when a number of psychoanalysts were seeking ways of using "Object Relations" to explain the uncharted intricacies of interpersonal relationships.

The distinction between the way in which Fairbairn, Klein, and Bion, three major contributing theorists to couple psychotherapy, respectively viewed the object relations system can be summarised as follows: Fairbairn's concern centred on an inner (unconscious) world of internalised bad objects, and their function in affecting relationships and forming the personality's structure; Klein's emphasis was on the externalisation (through projection) of painful and unwanted feelings, leading to a lack of good objects to build a coherent personality structure; and Bion focused on the impact of an inner world devoid of an object, which he saw as more devastating than one made up of bad or insufficient good ones.

Towards the end of Fairbairn's life, two formidable women in London, Enid Balint and Lily Pincus (Pincus, 1960), also extended object relations thinking about couples, developing the notion of the "couple fit." Fairbairn had no direct involvement in this, although, indirectly, his influence through Jock Sutherland and Henry Dicks was considerable.

Since his death in 1964, however, Fairbairn has risked being pushed into the footnotes of psychoanalytic literature, something that appears strange given all that he contributed to the establishment of the "Object Relations School." Sutherland hypothesises that he was ignored because some found his ideas too disturbing, but also largely because of the "hard intellectual work required" (Sutherland, 1989, p. 144). As Fairbairn's student, analysand, colleague, and biographer, Sutherland resolved to ensure that the canon of Fairbairn's work would not be forgotten. We have to thank him and other dedicated interpreters, including Dicks (1967), Harry Guntrip (1969), John Padel (1972), Jay Greenberg and Stephen Mitchell (1983), David Scharff and Jill Scharff (1991), Thomas Ogden (2010), and, most recently, Graham Clarke (Clarke & Scharff, 2014), for their persistence in this regard. Interestingly, the most recent authors are predominantly from North America; in the UK, Fairbairn is relatively unappreciated, like a "prophet in his own country."

Nevertheless, in considering the value of a modern-day application of Fairbairn's ideas, it is essential to question whether the theories of someone born in 1889, and who practised as a psychoanalyst with *individuals*, can possibly have continuing relevance for practitioners working with *couples*. David and Jill Scharff (2014, pp. 5–12), describing the theoretical components of psychodynamic couple therapy, put Fairbairn's model of psychic structure as a foundation stone. However, it may not necessarily be one which many practitioners can readily recall. Indeed, in order to assess the applicability of Fairbairn's ideas, it may be important to do so in the context of considering the needs of a "real live" couple whom we can hold in mind as we evaluate the insights of his theories.

As psychotherapists, we are continually challenged to say whether the theories we favour are evidence-based. Recently, many have looked instead for *practice-based evidence*. Sutherland liked to quote Kurt Lewin's aphorism that "There is nothing more practical than a good theory" (Lewin, 1952, p. 169). Certainly, we know that Fairbairn's theories were constructed out of closely observed clinical work; for him, the orthodoxy of Freud's thinking about drives was insufficient to account for the continuing effects of trauma experienced by his patients.

Putting practice first, therefore, I shall set out the main features of a case study, the identifying details of which are disguised, of a couple whom I shall call John and Simon. I will then summarise key Fairbairnian concepts most applicable to couple therapy before considering how they might be useful in understanding this couple's relationship.

## John and Simon

John and Simon have come at John's instigation to "sort out" Simon's request for some "time out" of their relationship. All previous discussions about it have ended in stalemate. We have agreed to a consultation process of three meetings, the second of which is now awaited. At our first meeting, I learn that John (aged 39 years) and Simon (aged 27 years) have been together for seven years and that John is keen, now that it is permitted, to get married. John describes himself as a "self-made man," with a successful IT business. Simon, recently qualified as an art therapist, is currently unemployed. John is perplexed and hurt to hear that Simon feels stifled and claustrophobic in the relationship and wants a "breathing space" to "be myself." How can this be, John reasons, because he has fully supported Simon to get a degree and to have therapy when he was depressed? Simon accepts this, saying that it is all his fault, but that he has sometimes felt afraid to stand up to John. John looks baffled.

John is the only child of separated parents. He has lost touch with his father, who was always emotionally distant, and who dismissed him when he came out at aged nineteen. His mother, chronically depressed for much of her life, is now in residential care with Alzheimer's disease. John says that he and Simon regard Simon's family as their family, and that they socialise a lot with one another.

Simon's father died when he was five years old; his mother is a nurse. He has two older sisters, both married with families. It emerges in the discussion that Simon felt vulnerable to bullying as he grew up, and that when he was "small" there was "a big upset" for which he blames himself. This was when his mother broke up with a boyfriend to whom Simon had felt very close.

Asking the couple what first drew them together, I learn that John admired Simon's youthful tenacity to overcome challenges. And he could dance! Simon found John strong and confident; he knew where he was going.

My impression of John is of a charming "businessman," used to getting his way. He is somewhat impatient with the expression of feelings that he does not understand. Simon, by contrast, is much quieter, somewhat boyish, and quite watchful of others' reactions, especially John's. He is much less certain and even fearful of speaking his mind. I find them both likeable, anxious to be accepted, but am left with a sense of underlying tensions and something "forced" about their presentation. I register some anxiety in myself about the risk of my own plain speaking and of asking leading questions, although I am puzzled about what it is that Simon is afraid of, which cannot be thought about or talked through.

## Key Fairbairnian concepts applicable in couple psychotherapy

Ronald Fairbairn was remarkable in the extraordinary scope of his thinking (Fairbairn, 1944). As well as making a special study of the schizoid personality, he wrote about trauma and its impact through early neglect, sexual and physical abuse, and through war; the structure of the personality and the stages of its development; the repression and return of bad objects; the significance of the family group in development; open and closed systems; the arts; and the treatment and rehabilitation of sexual offenders. For the purposes of this paper, I have grouped under five headings the concepts I consider most relevant for thinking about couple therapy.

### 1.   *The endopsychic structure of the personality*

This constitutes an essential starting point, because most of Fairbairn's theories stem from this premise, so much so, that near the very end of his life in 1963, "in response to many requests," he published *An Object Relations Theory of the Personality* (Fairbairn, 1963) as a clarifying "brief synopsis" of his theoretical position. Its seventeen points are listed like a credo, beginning with: "1. An ego is present from birth" and "2. Libido is a function of the ego." Fairbairn goes on to say that both the ego and the libido to which it is attached are fundamentally *object seeking* — from the very start of life the infant self is seeking a relationship with another. This simple assertion seems now to be uncontroversial, but at the time it was a departure from Freud's drive theory and from Klein's ideas about infant development. Thus, the infant self in relation with another was to be the foundation stone of Fairbairn's new complex personality structure.

The infant's search for a loving other is not always met sympathetically – he or she may be rejected. The mother or father (i.e., the object) may equally respond in an overly intrusive or tantalisingly seductive way. When the infant's reaching out for love has not been met with acceptance, Fairbairn believed that the first experience of anxiety is thus separation anxiety. The infant experiences the object's rejecting and confusing messages as *traumatic*. When the trauma is too painful and threatening, the infant deals defensively with the experience of unrequited love and resulting feelings of aggression and frustration by psychologically internalising the entire unsatisfactory experience. This means that aspects of the object (mother/father) and feelings about him or her are split off and repressed in the unconscious.

Because no infant-carer relationship is perfect, the experience of splitting of the ego in infancy is universal. Fairbairn saw it as the origin of schizoid phenomena. It follows that everyone is, in some degree, schizoid; the severity of this in the personality depends on how severely the infant has experienced rejection.

This can help us to understand John's difficulties. Arguably more schizoid than Simon, due to the way in which he was held at a distance by his father's rejection and from his mother's unavailability, it has left John less emotionally intelligent than Simon. Separation anxiety is, however, significant for them both. Fairbairn describes a process whereby the self, having split, is divided into three parts:

- A central (conscious) ego, attached to an ideal object or ego-ideal
- A repressed (unconscious) libidinal ego, attached to an exciting (or libidinal) object, and
- A repressed anti-libidinal ego, attached to a rejecting (or anti-libidinal) object. Fairbairn also called the "anti-libidinal ego" the "internal saboteur," which stresses its undermining role.

In this "inner" (unconscious) world, these split-off, repressed parts develop a stable, but *alterable*, relationship with one another. Sutherland (1989) sees them as a (libidinal) primitive need system that interacts with an (anti-libidinal) primitive control system. The libidinal need system expresses the infant's need to seek out his or her love object and is in constant tension with the anti-libidinal control system, which expresses the infant's desire to distance him or herself from his or her object. The vital developmental challenge in growing up is whether the central ego can manage these two subsystems, to ensure that neither one overrules the other. If the need system dominates, the individual will idealise others in a continual, but unrealisable, search for satisfaction. But if the control system takes charge, the individual will avoid relationships and sabotage that part of him or her that longs to be in one.

We can see how Fairbairn's description of the individual's relationship with a dynamic inner world made up of three interrelating parts provides a model that readily lends itself to explaining how human beings interact in wider close relationships – such as in couples, families, or groups. To achieve what is sometimes termed "inner peace," the individual growing up has to find — whether in parents, or family, or love relationships, or through psychotherapy — a satisfactory balance between the libidinal and anti-libidinal systems, thus ensuring there is less need for repression and greater scope for the central ego to make relationships. In the case of John and Simon, they are each too caught up in managing what had to be repressed to respond with the full acceptance that the other needs. Both have had good reason to doubt the safety of dependence. John's multiple rejections compel his continual pursuit to be Simon's dependable other; his libidinal ego seeks an unattainable lover. Simon, on the other hand, although longing for closeness with a father figure, mistrusts John's attention. His need to escape — his anti-libidinal ego — sabotages him from committing.

Why have they come for help now? They are now legally permitted to marry. Might gay marriages face higher societal expectations in matching up to an ideal? Both men are now experiencing a disturbing return of what has been repressed. External reality has brought to the surface John's awareness of how dependent this would-be self-made man is on a younger man; and how much he is drawn to and yearns for the love of someone who rejects him. It has also awakened Simon's awareness of his own fear of intimacy, particularly with a controlling adult.

## 2. *The moral defence*

The moral defence is formed in the process of repression. Fairbairn was struck by children's reluctance to remember experiences of abuse or neglect and concluded that this arose from a fear of reviving a relationship with a bad object that needed to be repressed. He noted that victims of maltreatment, whether by neglect, or physical or sexual abuse, preferred to see themselves as "bad" and those who had mistreated them as "good." He called this choice to keep them as good inner objects a "moral defence" because it was safer to be a "sinner in a world ruled by God than to live in a world ruled by the Devil" (Fairbairn, 1952, pp. 66–67). In essence, it was better to be guilty than helpless. We may conjecture also how this corresponds with Simon's need to see himself as the one responsible for everyone's unhappiness.

David Scharff also draws attention to how this defence helps explain why partners opt to stay in abusive relationships (Scharff, 2013). And we can see that it might have maintained the love–hate fit between Simon and John. Feeling guilt in preference to helplessness is triggered in Simon whenever there is a prospect of getting close to John, and every time he tries to break away. Simon felt guilty for having supposedly "caused" the break-up between his mother and her boyfriend. What is it about that experience that has had to be repressed? We may wonder whether it has been difficult to acknowledge that the boyfriend may have been sent away because he was grooming – perhaps abusing – Simon.

### 3. *Repression and the return of bad objects*

I want to explore further the potential for applying Fairbairn's ideas about repression in everyday work with couples. To do that it will first be important to acknowledge the work of Henry Dicks (1900–1977).

Working as a consultant psychiatrist at the Tavistock Clinic in London, Dicks was concerned to find a means of treating the epidemic in marriage and family breakdown happening in the post-war Britain of the mid-20th century. He was inspired by Fairbairn's ideas, that our capacity to relate to others begins in infancy; that psychopathology originates in the frustration of making relationships; and that our need for others and to feel needed by them is the basis of group life. Dicks's genius was to recognise that if he melded together Fairbairn's theories with Klein's concept of projective identification, it would create a practical basis for thinking about couple relationships. Thus was founded a new branch of psychoanalytic therapy — couple psychotherapy. In his seminal work, *Marital Tensions* (1967), Dicks set out hypotheses about couple relationships, based on the dynamics of idealisation, which he systematically and clinically tested to assess their validity in understanding couple relationship breakdown. Dicks had intuited a natural fit between Fairbairn's concept of the inherently object-seeking whole person ego and the couple as a unit made up of two instinctively object-seeking people. He realised that the relationship the couple creates develops a dynamic personality all of its own — a "joint marital personality," bound by "unconscious forces which flow between [them] forming bonds of a 'positive' and 'negative' kind, a love-hate involvement" (Dicks, 1967, p. 8). It is thanks to Dicks that in couple therapy the *relationship* is the patient — rather than one or each of the individual partners. While Dicks's thinking did contribute to the development of couple psychotherapy in the UK (Ruszczynski, 1993), his Fairbairnian concepts and his method were more fully elaborated in North America by John Zinner (1976) and by David Scharff and Jill Scharff (1991).

Repression is a defensive act in which bad, unsatisfactory, and even unsatisfying objects (i.e., experiences and the people they relate to) are internalised and put out of reach of awareness into the unconscious. It follows that the more that is repressed, the more impoverished the central ego becomes. An adult who is unconsciously preoccupied with managing an internal world which is disturbed by a forbidden or threatening object is somewhat handicapped when it comes to making a loving relationship because what is left to offer that relationship in his or her central ego has been rather depleted. Repressed objects do return to consciousness, however, in delusions, in breakdowns (whether constructive or damaging), in dreams, or in self-created failures. When they emerge, we might allow them to be usefully tried out in reality testing, or we may, with further repression, re-consign them to oblivion. Dicks saw the falling apart of marriages as an inevitable consequence of reality testing, when the return of the repressed has the potential to cause catastrophic damage to mutual idealisations.

Using this notion of the breach of mutual idealisations with regard to Simon and John, we can see that the threat of relationship breakdown — and the potential loss to John of Simon's family as well as his own — may force each of them to see that the strengths they first admired in one another in fact mask vulnerability. That vulnerability did not need to be acknowledged when John was the strong provider and Simon the grateful dependent. Now, however, Simon has had some therapy, and fear has also come to the surface. There may well be fear also of a deeper vulnerability, arising from the on-going sequelae of the traumas of rejection, abuse, and loss, and which is now marked by depression and loneliness. This fear is intolerable and cannot be spoken about.

### 4. *Open and closed systems*
In a late paper, Fairbairn (1958) describes the

> … struggle on the part of the patient to press-gang his relationship with the analyst into the closed system of the inner world through the agency of the transference, and [the] determination on the part of the analyst to effect a breach in this closed system and to provide conditions under which, in a setting of a therapeutic relationship, the patient may be induced to accept the open system of outer reality.
>
> (p. 385)

This idea illuminates for me the dynamics of working with couples who between them have created a closed system. Ostensibly, they ask for our help to address their difficulties, but all the while they resist attempts to allow an opening up to external realities. John and Simon have reported a situation of stalemate between them. My countertransference alerts me that asking probing questions might lead to unknown dangers and perhaps cause irreparable damage. Yet, if I were to go along with the strong message that we are there to get along well and please one another, I, too, would be drawn into their stuckness. My role is rather to tolerate being the outsider, offering an external view that opens up thinking and so tests their perceptions of reality.

More broadly speaking, perhaps the measure of the value of any psychoanalytic thinker is not to be found in the number of "truths" that they have nailed that stand for all time, but the degree to which they inspire new insights. It is as if when reading them they invite us into an open system. This kind of sharing enables practitioners to continue thinking, especially when we feel we are under fire, as when patients try to dragoon us into their closed system.

### 5.  *The development of dependence*

Fairbairn saw development as a journey of personal growth through-out which dependence on relationships with others is essential. Starting out from the complete dependence of the baby, the journey ideally culminates in an adult's mature dependence. He says that in mature dependence, the adult can appreciate "not that the libidinal attitude is essentially genital [as in infancy], but that the genital attitude is essentially libidinal" (Fairbairn, 1952, p. 32). To achieve a state of adult genitality, the individual has to have worked through the difficulties of loving and being loved in infancy, so that in adulthood it feels possible to let go a relationship that proves unsatisfactory. "The more mature a relationship, the less it is characterised by primary identification … in favour of relationships with differentiated objects" (p. 42). For Fairbairn, dependence on parents is therefore gradually widened out to a point that it is ultimately rested in culture and society. It may be very instructive to think about how couple relationships fit into a pic-ture of development towards mature dependence. Couples like John and Simon speak to us of many partners' resistance to allowing that kind of growth in one another.

## Conclusion

In re-finding Fairbairn and weighing up his overall contribution, we can observe someone who strove hard to devise theories that would serve his patients. What comes across in reading him, in addition to his astute intellect, is his essential humanity and his enormous concern for people. He believed that the determining factor in the success of any treatment was the therapist's ability to make a relationship with his or her patient. He was also open to revising his ideas. While it is clear that Fairbairn did not have all the answers to the problems that he identified (social attitudes, notably those towards homosexuality, have since markedly changed), he pursued his work until his death, leaving a legacy that could be developed and applied by others.

In this exploration of the potential application of some of Fairbairn's key concepts, my aim has been to refresh a familiarity with Fairbairn's work the better to assess whether it still offers couple therapists resources to face current therapeutic challenges. While Fairbairn was not writing directly about couple psychotherapy, in my view, his observations remain insightful because they are relationally based. Although his patients were all individuals, he saw them as members of social groups – families or couples. So, if nowadays, when reading Fairbairn, we gain an insight into one partner's difficulties (e.g., moral defence), we are prompted to ask what part it plays in the couple fit. Today's couples present difficulties of ever-increasing complexity and intractability – they are not just the "worried well." Marriage may be less common, but the desire to couple remains strong. Perhaps, compared with previous generations, today's couples have lower expectations that their relationship will outlive disillusionment. Can a couple's relationship really be the dependable container or medium in which together they might successfully work out the conflicts that were unresolved when they were growing up? Maybe it could, with the help of a therapist who can model open-mindedness. Against the backdrop of hope vs. disillusionment, couples who seek help have often survived traumas, the trauma of childhood sexual, physical, and emotional abuse, or of military conflict, or of neglect and abandonment. They may also be burdened by the fallout from aggression, personality disorder, mental illness, and addictions. While this characterisation seems all too common today, sadly, as I have conveyed, it would also have sounded depressingly familiar to both Fairbairn and Dicks.

In discussing Fairbairn's relevance today, I have raised questions about the relationship between theory and practice. We may want to debate how our allegiance to a particular set of theories actually influences our practice. It might be claimed that surely our choice of theoretical stance affects our understanding of our countertransference and how we should frame our interpretations. We may still be uncertain, however, as to what is *mutative* when it comes to choosing the appropriate technique. When should we give voice to our counter-transference? Are our interpretations really as significant as the relationship we create in the threesome? Reading Fairbairn, however, confirms for me that a good grounding in theory helps to contain the therapist. Containment results in there being less temptation to respond to the countertransference through enactments and so be recruited into the couple's closed system. Furthermore, my clinical experience endorses that of Fairbairn, in suggesting that, ultimately, the degree to which we can hope to offer troubled couples containment is going to depend both on our capacities to relate to them, and on our willingness to be open to new ways of thinking, some of which may need to be rediscovered from the past.

## References

Barker, P.M.W. (1996). *The regeneration trilogy*. London: Viking Books.

Clarke, G.S. & Scharff, D.E. (2014). *Fairbairn and the object relations tradition*. London: Karnac.

Dicks, H.V. (1967). *Marital tensions*. London: Routledge.

Fairbairn, W.R.D. (1931). Features in the analysis of a patient with a physical genital abnormality. In: *Psychoanalytic studies of the personality* (pp. 197–222). London: Tavistock.

Fairbairn, W.R.D. (1944). Endopsychic structure considered in terms of object-relationships. *International Journal of Psycho-Analysis*, 25, 70–73.

Fairbairn, W.R.D. (1952). *Psychoanalytic studies of the personality*. London: Tavistock.

Fairbairn, W.R.D. (1958). On the nature and aims of psycho-analytical treatment. *International Journal of Psycho-Analysis*, 39(5), 374–385.

Fairbairn, W.R.D. (1963). Synopsis of an object relations theory of the personality. *International Journal of Psycho-Analysis*, 44, 224–225.

Greenberg, J. & Mitchell, S. (1983). *Object relations in psychoanalytic theory*. Cambridge, MA: Harvard University Press.

Guntrip, H. (1969). *Schizoid phenomena, object relations and the self*. New York: International Universities Press.

Lewin, K. (1952). *Field theory in social science*. London: Tavistock.

Ogden, T.H. (2010). Why read Fairbairn? *International Journal of Psychoanalysis*, 91, 101–108.

Padel, J. (1972). The contribution of W.R.D. Fairbairn to psychoanalytic theory and practice. *Bulletin of the European Psycho-Analytic Federation*, 2, 13–26.

Pincus, L. (Ed.). (1960). *Marriage: Studies in emotional conflict and growth*. London: Institute of Marital Studies.

Ruszczynski, S.J. (Ed.). (1993). *Psychotherapy with couples*. London: Karnac.

Scharff, D.E. (2013). Aggression in couples: An object relations primer. *Couple and Family Psychoanalysis*, 3(1), 47–60.

Scharff, D.E. & Scharff, J.S. (1991). *Object relations couple therapy*. Northvale, NJ: Jason Aronson.

Scharff, D.E. & Scharff, J.S. (Eds.). (2014). *Psychoanalytic couple therapy*. London: Karnac.

Sutherland, J.D. (1989). *Fairbairn's journey into the interior*. London: Free Association Books.

Zinner, J. (1976). The implications of projective identification for marital interaction. In H. Grunebaum & J. Christ (Eds.), *Contemporary marriage structure, dynamics and therapy* (pp. 293–308). Boston, MA: Little Brown.

## Chapter 12

# Discussion of "Lost – and found – in translation"

## Do Ronald Fairbairn's ideas still speak usefully to 21st-century couple therapists?

*Leora Benioff*

Molly Ludlam starts right off, lucidly – and accurately – presenting Fairbairn as the visionary father of Object Relations theory whose seminal contribution to psychoanalytic theory has been largely disregarded, particularly in Kleinian circles. Fairbairn was born and lived in Scotland, 400 miles away from the intensely generative and regressive forces of the psychoanalytic community of mid-20th-century London. Surmising that he also may have further distanced himself by presenting his original thinking in highly technical – sometimes impenetrable – abstract language, Ludlam articulately provides us with a clear translation of Fairbairn's ideas and then further brings his work to life with her discussion of the usefulness of his ideas in contemporary couple psychoanalytic psychotherapy.

Inspired by Ludlam's study, I immersed myself in Fairbairn's ideas. My experience of this immersion was surprising to me. Unlike many other psychoanalytic writers, his work did not beckon me in. As Ludlam noted, his writing seems cold, distant, and saturated. But the more I got past the writing and lived with his ideas while I worked, the more these ideas came to life in the very human struggles of the couples I was seeing. Now, I would like to describe what happens when I bring Fairbairn into the consulting room, and where it takes my thinking on working with couples.

As psychoanalysts, we welcome our patients' intense – sometimes seemingly one-dimensional and limited – views of us, and call this "the transference." We believe this transference powerfully brings to life the emotional truth of their experience. An attempt to talk patients out of this experience, to explain to them why their views of us are distorted, only partially true, or too one-sided, would be strange and counter-productive.

DOI: 10.4324/9781003265023-12

Yet, when treating couples, as analytic therapists, we often find our-selves doing just that. Faced with someone who is deeply pained by feeling misperceived and mischaracterised by his or her partner, and convinced that this misrecognition is with malignant intention, we feel a pressure to help the "misperceiving" and "distorting" partner shift his or her view of the other – perhaps by disentangling past relation-ships from present, and hoping to create conditions for a more realis-tic view. This rarely works. It is in opposition to what we come to know as psychoanalysts: the life goes out of a treatment when we attempt to convince people not to feel, think, or believe what they feel, think, or believe.

Central to Fairbairn's thinking is that the young child, completely vulnerable and dependent, must survive by maintaining a connection to the parent (usually the mother) at any cost. The child who suffers insufficient or problematic contact and care (in reality, every child at some point) internalises the parent in particular ways, sorting out and creating one-sided internal characters that represent the unsatisfac-tory components of his or her experiences. In these circumstances, there is a hungry, rejected, internal character who is addictively con-nected to an exciting, out-of-reach, tantalising character. There is a ruminative, angry, victimised character attached to a cruel, rejecting, character. All these characters are developed in an unconscious, inter-nal split-off world as a way of trying to fix the connection to a disap-pointing and problematic caregiver. Adult couple relationships powerfully bring to life the deep structures of these attachments to unresolved, unsatisfying, one-sided characters and relationships, and the immense energy and gravitational pull they evince. Poignantly, much of couple conflict is rooted in the painful desperation of a small child trying to stay psychologically alive and connected in the face of unmet needs.

With Fairbairn, and these intense inner objects and dynamics in mind, I came to understand much more deeply and fully the very frequent need of one or both members of a couple to perceive and experience the other in a rigidly negative and stereotyped manner. Fairbairn (1944, 1958) describes how a patient can "press-gang" the analyst to accept this rigid internal orthodoxy – and the same dynamic also happens with a life partner. Fairbairn's description of the inner world – replete with its ensemble of one-sided, intense characters living out repetitive themes and fixed interpersonal "set pieces" – lends itself to couple therapy by helping us identify the intense emotions that shape these rigid one-sided emotional experiences in couple relationships. As Ludlam says,

> This idea illuminates for me the dynamics of working with couples who between them have created a closed system. Ostensibly, they ask for our help to address their difficulties, but all the while they resist attempts to allow an opening up to external realities.

> (this volume, p. 151)

The crucial question in couple therapy is how to modify a closed system. There needs to be some way for people to modify their inner objects and to perceive new external objects. Fairbairn (1958) believes that the way into a closed system is through the introduction of a new, good object (the analyst). Yet, he never satisfactorily explains how a new object can be introduced and accepted, which is the very problem with a closed system – all new objects are seen as old. I am suggesting here that one important aspect of transforming a closed system into a more open system is to have one's inner world – with its undiluted and distorted characters dominating one's emotional experience – known, understood, and somehow accepted by one's partner.

Some current post-Bionian psychoanalytic ideas (Ferro, 2002; Ogden, 2016) posit that it's necessary to have one's inner world lived out, as a waking dream, so that it can be known, understood, and digested. I wonder if we could continue our current 21st-century thinking based on Bion and post-Bion field theory – which sees life as a constant waking dream – to understand as couple psychotherapists this relationship of internal to external objects lived out in our consulting rooms. In order to process experience, change, and grow, it's important that our inner lives be represented both in our own minds and in the minds of the people whom we rely on. As James Fisher (1999) so eloquently explains, couple stories can be seen as dreams that illuminate people's internal object worlds and painful emotional experiences, dreams that have to be known by being lived through. Fairbairn, as a phenomenologist of these inner worlds, helps us much more fully understand the unconscious components of our experience in relationships, and thus gives a shape to emotional experience such that it can be digested and understood, and optimally, transformed.

Years ago, I worked with a couple whom I shall call Richard and Dina. The work seemed to be developing well, with more room for thoughtful response to one another and less incendiary conflict. Richard was able to recognise the personal importance of his mother's severe postpartum depression after the birth of a younger sibling. A seemingly benign comment, however, about a brief relationship Dina had had with another man many years before they met greatly upset Richard. Although usually calm and easy-going, Richard was overcome with anxiety. He was utterly sure that Dina found this man more desirable and far more exciting. He remained distraught, although he could not cite anything Dina had said or done that showed she preferred the other man. Dina's efforts to assure Richard of his desirability did not calm him down but further inflamed and upset him. My attempts to point out that he seemed to be intent upon viewing himself as insufficiently attractive in Dina's eyes also didn't help. He clung to his idea as if his life depended upon it. And, from Fairbairn's point of view, his life did depend on it – his internal life. Richard's intransient dedication to see his relationship with Dina as if it were his relationship with his rejecting, depressed mother would have had everything to do with the internal reality he created in his struggle for emotional survival. Paradoxically, the liveliest and potentially expansive indications of emotional truth in couple relationships are just these expressions of experiencing the other in rigid, unrealistically one-sided, ways, and the fierce clinging to these one-dimensional views.

I am reminded of another couple, Howard and Everett, who struggled despite a clear and sound commitment to one another. At 5:30 one morning, Howard went to the gym without telling Everett. Everett woke to find himself alone. Because Howard had never before left without telling him, he was convinced that Howard had left him, never to return. In the couple psychotherapy, Howard volubly protested that he hadn't and never would leave him. Everett rejected the therapist's suggestion that even though Howard had only left to go to the gym, Everett nevertheless had a painful experience of being abandoned. Everett was intent upon convincing Howard and the therapist that he actually had been left for good. The evidence of this, according to Everett, was Howard's basic tendency to abandon. As with the previous vignette, Everett felt painfully misunderstood when the therapist and Howard attempted to convince him to adopt a more "realistic" view.

For Everett, something crucial needed to happen in order for him to feel content living with the abandoning other. Everett didn't want Howard to convince him that his intentions were good. Rather, he wanted Howard to recognise that to abandon him was simply a fixed aspect of his character – that he was an abandoner. For Howard to endorse this view of himself – as if he were a character in a cartoon – seemed far more important to Everett's peace of mind than the fact that Howard stayed put and continued to be emotionally engaged with Everett. For Howard to accept his role as the abandoning loved one was to see Everett, as he so deeply needed to be seen – as the abandoned, unloved one.

What Everett wanted from Howard is not that unusual. There is a particular state of mind in which a yearning exists for one's inner stereotyped aspects of their mind to be known, validated, and accepted. This desire is strangely accompanied by an unquestioned acceptance of the relationship and the other as is. What seems important is that the other accepts this distorted characterisation of oneself because it is experienced as one's true and native self. If this can happen, the aggrieved can move on, feeling recognised and loved. As with the transference in individual treatment, the aggrieved member of the couple in treatment needs first to have their negative experiences of their partner explored and validated, rather than corrected.

Fairbairn's ideas suggest that in a schizoid state, with the defences necessary to cope with painful early relationships, it is crucial to maintain a completely negative experience of some aspects of a current, real-life, loved one, so that one can keep intact an inner world of compartmentalised, one-sided inner objects. Fairbairn reminds us that this inner structure – of yearning and angry feelings and qualities being kept split off from each other by dissociation – is fundamental to the structure of the personality, albeit a depleted and diminished one. This structure is also, paradoxically, very crucial to keeping the hope alive that one can fix deeply disappointing inner objects and relations. The paradox is that the structure of overly one-sided perceptions and experiences, which seems to be a cause of disappointing and disturbing relations, is actually an attempt to preserve and repair relationships.

Closely related to one or both partners' stranglehold on their internal worlds – at the expense of allowing the fresh air and sunlight of the reality of the external world – is the refusal of ambivalence, and the seeming incapacity to experience the mingled yarn of love and the hate. This intolerance of ambivalence is one of the hallmarks of an unhappy couple. Fairbairn's ideas come into play in our thinking about these couples, as they rest on the concept that bad feelings must be kept locked up and completely separated from the yearning, tender feelings, and thus must never be diminished or ameliorated. The psychological function of this splitting defence is to avoid ambivalence. For the analytic therapist, the experience of ambivalence is a developmental achievement. As Ogden (2010) says,

> For Fairbairn, the most difficult and most psychically formative psychological problem that the infant or child faces is the dilemma that arises when he experiences his mother (upon whom he is utterly dependent) as both loving and accepting of his love, and unloving and rejecting of his love.
>
> (p. 102)

Hence, ways of coping with unbearable pressures in childhood lead to a problematic inability to deal with complexity and an inability to have mixed feelings and perceptions in adult love relationships. The more extreme the splitting, the more people are, desperately and unconsciously, protecting some version of their love and internalised objects as "good." This desperation is a painful reminder that the bad and negative experiences of each other must be treated with sympathy and tender respect in couple treatment.

Fairbairn (1952) compellingly describes an idealising defence, what he calls "the moral defence," in which all guilt must lie with the self, not the other, in order to protect the sense of the possibility of a good object. This is an extremely useful idea in individual and couple therapy, as we track the extreme flips between accusations and self-blame that can occur rapidly in a couple. Frequently, it is startlingly clear that at times people cannot tolerate seeing their partners at fault. According to Fairbairn, this realistic perception would leave them in a world of bad objects, without hope. But Fairbairn's ideas also can help us understand the opposite phenomenon, a clinical fact commonly experienced by couple therapists, the intense attachment to a perception of the partner as a bad (disappointing, rejecting, engulfing, oblivious) object.

Perhaps, the first order is to allow one partner to experience the other as a particular kind of completely bad object, because this is how they need to be known. The inner world of intense, one-sided, and stereotyped relationships cannot be known and digested unless it is lived with. When working with couples, it is essential that the bad inner characters, and the qualities of relating to them, be fully explored. This also gives people the chance to heal, to translate their inner worlds into found experience. So, when thinking about patients who need to have their negative experiences of their partners validated and explored, rather than deconstructed and disproved, perhaps we can understand this as an essential first stage in their quest to be understood and helped to love.

There is a constant dialectic in couple psychotherapy between a therapeutic stance of accepting and mirroring these negative relational emotional experiences on the one hand, and interpreting and confronting splitting and projection on the other. When the therapist, as a representative from the external world, enters into the couple's complaints about each other, and the bad characters they experience each other as, this can help each of them disentangle the current experiences from their internal and past relations. However, as I have described, a locked-in pattern commonly emerges when the couple relate to each other's dissociated, and split off, internal objects. When members of a couple enact something emotionally similar to their dissociated and one-dimensional unconscious internal objects, it is painful, but magnetically compelling to them. Invariably, it sticks like hot glue when one person engages with another who enacts some familiar feature of his or her own inner world. In these instances, what appears to be a small similarity to the negative internal object can be experienced as the entire negative internal object. Fairbairn (1943) wonderfully describes in terms of patients with what we would now speak about as having "combat-related PTSD":

> An unconscious situation involving internalized bad objects is liable to be activated by any situation in outer reality conforming to a pattern which renders it emotionally significant in light of the unconscious situation. It is for this reason that the psychoneurotic soldier cannot bear to be shouted at by the sergeant major and cannot bear to eat army food. For in his eyes every word of command is equivalent to assault, and every spoonful of greasy stew is a drop of poison from the breast of a malevolent mother.
>
> (p. 81)

I find this dynamic very powerful to observe as it is something we see in our daily work with couples. Slight difficulties become intolerable and insurmountable – a small shift in tone, a small difference in taste or capacity to accommodate suddenly turns the relation into one of persecution and rejection. Due to dissociation and internal splitting, a negative object is the only one present in that moment. So, a partner often seems worse than he or she is, a part is mistaken for the whole, as one-dimensional and persecutory. It is the couple therapist's job to help the partners tolerate and become curious about these negative experiences that are due to their inner worlds combining with their defensive proclivities and actions. At the same time, the therapist must slowly help them see the difference between their perception/emotional experience of the partner and their partner's own, complex, mixed intentions. This eventually helps create a relational space between inner and outer experience, where each member of the couple can be seen as both a bad object, and as an external, tender, and vulnerable other.

As the two vignettes above illustrate, couple therapists frequently have the experience that confronting a member of a couple with evidence that their partner is not as bad as they had believed, does not provide relief. In fact, the partner can become furious, feel misunderstood, and double down on efforts to convince everyone in the room of their true disappointing nature. This is a common cause of intense couple fights. The partner perceived as bad will become defensive and argumentative, trying to convince the other of his or her benign and misperceived intentions. As we all know, these fights go nowhere. But why should this be? One would assume that people would be so relieved and happy to find out that their partners are not rejecting them, that they actually do have them in mind, and are not full of dislike, abandonment, or hatred.

In such cases, in order to maintain an inner world of one-sided characters and interactions, it seems imperative for an aggrieved partner to maintain a completely negative experience of some aspects of the current loved one. So, what does a couple therapist do in situations entrenched with endopsychic structures? Using Fairbairn (1944, 1952, 1958), and Ogden's (2010) "translation" of Fairbairn, the couple therapist needs to work with both partners towards a diminution:

> ... of the intensity of the feelings of resentment, addictive love, contempt, primitive dependence, disillusionment, and so on that bind the split off, repressed sub-organizations of the self to one another.
>
> (p. 114)

Lessening the inner bind in one or both partners, allows for a fuller bond with each other as external, real, and separate objects. Ogden (2010), in writing about Fairbairn, says that true psychological growth comes about by a patient's

> ... genuine acceptance of himself and, by extension, acceptance of others. That acceptance is achieved by ... coming to terms with the full range of aspects of oneself, including one's disturbing, infantile, split off identifications with one's unloving, unaccepting mother [or his/her partner]. Psychological change of this sort creates the possibility of discovering a world of people and experiences that exists outside of oneself, a world in which ... one feels no compulsion to transform the realities of one's human relationships into something other than what they are, i.e. to change oneself or "the object" (who is now a whole and separate subject) into other people. It is also a world in which one can learn from one's experience with other people because those experiences are no longer dominated by projections of static internal object relationships.
>
> (p. 114)

The title of Molly Ludlam's chapter eloquently captures this transformation: "Lost – and found – in translation." Parts of the self are compartmentalised and buried, due to deeply painful and disappointing early relations. They are found again in intimate relations and reappear as one-dimensional characters acting out a scripted drama. The intimate partner can find them, now with an understanding of the inner world of his or her partner. But it is up to the couple therapist to translate these characters into a language of understanding and intimacy, rather than one of persecution and malignant misunderstanding. It is up to the couple therapist to create the conditions for the psychological work that will help the couple translate these characters into a fuller, more realistic self, an experience with both good and bad feelings about oneself and their partner. For all of us, the most basic human need and source of emotional vitality is to be fully known and loved, and this can get so easily thrown off track and impede our ability to love others and have that love received.

# References

Fairbairn, W.R. (1943). The repression and the return of bad objects (with special reference to the "war neuroses"). In *Psychoanalytic studies of the personality* (pp. 28–58). London: Routledge and Kegan Paul.

Fairbairn, W.R. (1944). Endopsychic structure considered in terms of object relationships. In *Psychoanalytic studies of the personality* (pp. 82–132). London: Routledge and Kegan Paul.

Fairbairn, W.R. (1952). *An object relations theory of the personality.* London: Routledge and Kegan Paul.

Fairbairn, W.R. (1958). On the nature and aims of psychoanalytical treatment. *International Journal of Psychoanalysis,* 39: 374–385.

Ferro, A. (2002). *In the Analyst's consulting room.* New York: Taylor and Francis, Inc.

Fisher, J. (1999). *The uninvited guest: Emerging from narcissism towards marriage.* London: Karnac Books.

Ogden, T.H. (2010). Why read Fairbairn? *International Journal of Psychoanalysis,* 91, 101–118.

Ogden, T.H. (2016). *Reclaiming unlived life: Experiences in psychoanalysis.* London: Routledge.

Chapter 13

# Approaching couples through the lens of Link Theory

*Monica Vorchheimer*

How is it that the members of a couple fail to understand each other? What happens when they lose their capacities to make themselves understandable or to achieve an understanding of their partner? Why is this difficulty often felt to be so disappointing, even catastrophic? And why, during these times, isn't love enough? Many couples do not view these types of difficulties in understanding one another as part of the normal vicissitudes of ordinary life. Rather, they regard it as a kind of malformation, something that should never occur. Moreover, when they feel that they no longer understand each other, one or both of them usually presumes that it is the partner who is in the wrong. This type of presentation is frequently encountered in couple psychotherapy and poses particular concerns for those who work with couples.

This paper outlines some of the key theoretical and clinical concepts stemming from Link Theory, an approach that can be used to provide valuable tools for clinicians and shed light on these types of problems. Link Theory, developed in Latin America over the last fifty years, has greatly influenced the widespread interest and practice of psychoanalysis with couples and families in Argentina and has increasingly generated interest across the world.

## New ideas

Traditional psychoanalytic theory understands love relationships as the effect of reciprocal projective identifications pari passu, an extension of individual analysis. It was only later that the psychic effects of being part of a relationship were also recognised as a new source of subjectivity. This discovery constitutes an important change in psychoanalytic tradition, which has hitherto focused primarily on internal

DOI: 10.4324/9781003265023-13

reality and the world of object representations. Link Theory introduces external reality – the "other" of the relationship – into the corpus of psychoanalytic theory and practice and stresses the relevance
of the effects of the presence of the object, not only of its absence. The
presence of the other, and its psychic effects on the constitution of the
mind. has previously been underestimated. By considering the other
(the object of the link) as merely a character, or as an inhabitant of
unconscious phantasy in the internal world, its significance has been
downplayed (Hobsbawm & Ranger, 1983).

Psychoanalysis has a rich tradition grounded in a metapsychology of
repetition. Instincts (drives), repetition compulsion, trauma, après
coup, transference, dreamlife, infantile sexuality, and even love have
been understood in terms of the theory of repetition. In contrast, Link
Theory brings that which is new into the picture. It offers the idea that
subjects are shaped not only by their historical relationship with the
body ego and the drives. but also by their links with others and their
social environment (Berenstein, 2001a; Berenstein, 2001b; Berenstein,
2012). From this standpoint, the link can be seen as a new metapsycho-
logical object that presents a "demand for psychic work" (Moguillansky
and Seiguer, 1996). This demand for psychic work arises from the fact
of belonging to the link and requires doing something with the other,
with the presence of the other, and with the meanings that are derived
from the other. This goes beyond the interplay of projective identifications and involves thinking about the consequences of being part of a
relationship itself, something the individual subjects cannot fully know
because they cannot be aware of their singular unconscious determinations. Nor can they be aware of the determinations which stem from the
link they belong to as well. Subjects in the link must make room for the
presence of the other as an other and, in this way, manage the novelty
involved in being part of a link. The subject is thus conceived as being
both a subject of the unconscious and a subject of the link that presents
a demand for psychic work. The constitution of identity is, therefore, a
biphasic process that implies both the internalisation of objects through
identifications and an identificatory imposition coming from the link.

## The couple as the use of a plural

People typically refer to the couple in the plural, as "we," alluding to
the set to which they feel they belong. "Set" is a term borrowed from

set theory, a branch of mathematics, used to describe a collection of elements. In the context of couples, the set refers to a collection of internal and external objects that represent the togetherness of the couple, that which they feel and recollect.

Importantly, the use of the plural reveals a number of things. The plural provides materiality to the feeling of belonging to that set and is evident in formulations such as. "It is good for us as a couple to go out once a week …" or; "We yell when we argue, which is a burden for us." The couple equates this emotional experience to a natural experience, a reality. The representation underlying these enunciations substantiates a phantasy that helps create a sense of identity. It is not only as an individual self-identity but, more importantly, the identity of the togetherness of the couple. As with every identity, the identity of the couple is conceived of as everlasting and as a source of security. This is the main reason why the members of the couple defend it forcefully and with an attitude of certainty.

The members of the couple consider that the "we" (the set) has the status of a real thing. It is something natural, almost tangible. Moreover, the "we," the plural itself, becomes a reality, making people assume with conviction that they can apprehend the existence of that reality. This presupposes that there is only one reality and that when they speak about it, they are speaking about a true reality, a totalising reality, a reality that can be captured in words. They ignore the fact that the couple is nothing but an emotional experience, neither accessible through words, nor through the senses. From a psychoanalytic point of view, the "we," like the unconscious, has no materiality.

This misconception about being able to see the couple as if it were a reality is not tempered by the use of language. The fact that words have multiple meanings, some of which are not necessarily known to participants in the conversation, contributes to the proliferation of misunderstandings. While we accept that words are polysemic, such acceptance is often only intellectual. Although a person may say, "This is just my point of view" to indicate that they are avoiding absolute fundamentalist views, this is easier said than meant. We are seldom aware of how partial our views are. Being a subject of an (emotional) experience is incompatible with being an impartial witness to that experience. We can only have partial versions, perspectives that cannot grasp the experience as a totality.

Operating in a state of fundamentalist views inevitably leads to misunderstandings. It is common to see partners interpret misunderstandings as lies and accuse each other of not telling the truth. The act of seeing differently is thereby considered foreign to the truth of the matter. Here are some examples of these types of interactions:

"Don't lie! Tell her how things really happened."
"It's you who aren't telling the truth! I didn't say that!"
"You did say it. That's exactly what happened."
"It wasn't like that at all!

These examples illustrate how the members of a couple think that they are able to visualise the set they belong to but are oblivious to the fact that they have only partial vision. They cannot imagine that they do not see what they do not see. Both think that the speaker can see the couple from an overall perspective, and when they speak about the couple, they believe they have the ability to see the couple as a whole, to fully understand what is going on. This is where the breakdown in the couple occurs.

## A common beginning

JOHN: The reason we're here is that we have conflicts, and we have a hard time communicating. We don't understand each other anymore. She says what she thinks, how she sees things, and I say how I see them, and we don't agree, and we end up raising our voices, especially me. She reacts, she says things, and everything ends in an argument. She brought up the idea of going into therapy, and it seemed okay to me.

MARY: The thing is that we start talking about something, and anything I say he takes badly. If I say, "That sweater is old fashioned," he sees it as a criticism. Maybe I don't say it in the best way, but he takes everything badly, he gets defensive. And there is no way to develop a coherent conversation about anything: the kids, money, school. There is a lot of tension. We can't maintain a normal dialogue or say anything without feeling we are criticizing each other. I feel he misunderstands what I say, and I probably misunderstand what he says, too.

Those who are familiar with couple psychotherapy might recognise this beginning of a session as quite typical. As often happens, John and Mary believe that they have a communication problem that they should not have. They suffer because they believe they should not have this problem. They are both talking about what "the thing" is, what is happening to them, what the reason or the source of their conflicts and discontent is. The fact of having different explanations for "the thing" increases the pain and anxiety of the failed encounter. Their difference is painfully experienced as the evidence of the loss of something which they assume they once (previously) had – a meeting with the other that represented the set to which they belonged. They presume there previously existed such an ideal encounter with the other and that it has now vanished.

In trying to explain what the problem is in this way, as many couples do, John and Mary are trying to do something they believe is possible, but it is impossible. They are trying to capture something that they feel they have lost or are losing. When they look for reasons or try to identify what is going on, they are trying to retrieve something as if it were a concrete "thing." Yet, they ignore that this is nothing but a representation, an aspect of the link as something that is thought to be tangible. They ignore that the thing they are trying to grasp is an emotional "thing" that cannot be apprehended by the senses. However, when they seek to find this, they try to provide substance, materiality to that something, the couple-set, which has very little substance or consistency. Nonetheless, this representation of togetherness is not experienced as a representation, but as the thing in itself. Hence, one of the difficulties that all couples tend to have in thinking of themselves is related to the fallacy of considering the couple to be a material reality. But if the couple is not a "real thing," what is it?

## The need for representation: the narcissistic foundation of couples

Freud (1914) suggested that the individual ego develops from the initial chaos of drives and moves towards a unified representation of the self (primary narcissism). This development is regardless of how imaginary this representation might be. Similarly, the reference to the "we" of the couple denotes the representation of a set – a unity that is also an imaginary representation. We do not need to assign this representation a spatial location; it is enough for the partners to believe in its existence.

While being part of a couple, or belonging to a set, people believe that Paradise, a narcissistic state, exists or that it existed in their history (Aulagnier, 2015). The infantile ideal ego is thought to have possessed perfection, inherited and displaced from the original Paradise of narcissism. Similarly, the illusion of love contains an idealised belief, an ideal set where adversities can be overcome as a result of love and that, while loving, infinity can be reached, and all dreams will be fulfilled. A phantasy of perfection hovers over couples in love, concealing defects, incompleteness, and differences. Similar to Freud's idea of "His Majesty the Baby," it could be said that couples in love imagine their own Paradise: "Our Majesty the We." In the same way that parents negate death through the phantasy of the generational continuity with their baby, love negates finitude through the imagined dimension of eternity: love will last forever.

I am suggesting that sets can be conceived as being constituted in the same way as Freud's idea of original narcissism. The representation of the set as a "we" provides partners with a sense of stability and identity and serves to deny the transience of emotionality. The emotional experience of belonging to the set lies beyond the grasp of the external senses and can only be experienced. It happens and disappears; it happens again and soon vanishes; it is evanescent, transient. However, as part of a link, we need this to be fixed in order to deny its transience. When this type of representation of the link as a unity – as a narcissistic whole – works, it is mute. In a psychoanalytic treatment, this representation can only be inferred from the joint productions of those participating in that set, just as Freud himself inferred the phantasies underlying narcissism from clinical phenomena.

The feeling of togetherness in the couple is supported by their creation of a fusional totality, the phantasy of a completeness that is heir to the original narcissistic foundation of the couple. Conversely, when this representation that encompasses them both cannot be constructed, they experience a feeling of loss, and this loss feels real to the couple – it is the loss of the set itself.

## Paradise: origin as illusion

Just as the theory of narcissism was born out of Freud's need to create a logical consistency to the ontogenesis of the psyche, we can reconstruct the couple's mythical foundation – the origin, the ontogenesis of that set. Sometimes partners speak about this origin explicitly, and are so enthusiastic about their beginnings, that it seems as if that first passionate encounter is happening again, right as they speak about it. They are describing an invention of an identity (every identity is an invention) that makes them believe in a continuity of the existence of the set, a "continuous we" that remains stable beyond their encounters. When they are surrounded by this atmospheric sense of falling in love again, like the first time, they assume that the experience is the same for both of them. It is an identity that is an invention, but is not experienced as such by the couple. They think of it as an actual fact, and this gives their origin great significance. They believe everything started in Paradise. They believe in magic!

It is my assumption, not the couple's, that the experience of falling in love is the effect of an illusory belief that they share the same representation, the same illusion – a phantasy of fusion that extols similarities and coincidences through sameness, or by accepting differences only when they can constitute complementarities. The result is a total identity, an identity of a totality, of completeness, a "we." The partners think they have had a magic encounter precisely because they believe that they both have had the same experience simultaneously. It is this illusion of having the same illusion that lends the paradisiacal quality of magic to the feeling of being in love.

This type of an illusion of a shared belief with a partner produces an identity for the set and reunites the partners through an illusion similar to early narcissism, bringing back together that which was previously disaggregated. Our Majesty the We! The resulting identity derives from the illusion that the encounter has created something exceptional, lasting, and stable. Differences are disavowed and what is alien is seen as not belonging to the "we." There is no room in this illusion to imagine that each partner is an other.

This idea of the origin of the couple – as creating the illusion of a shared representation of the couple – can be understood, metapsychologically, as a foundational myth that helps the couple feel they are truly together. It should be stressed here that each representation of the set is an individual representation, although we use the plural to refer to it. The myth can only be expressed through the subjectivity of the individual. The need to assume that it is a shared reality is the result of the narcissistic foundation of the couple, the phantasy that has brought two subjectivities together. Moreover, lovers fall in love not only with each other but also with this representation. It is worth recalling how often we hear that lovers are in love with love; they are in love with the representation that they imagine they share. They are in love with the set represented in this illusion of having the same illusion. It is as if they could identify with the gaze of a third eye that watches this couple in love.

## The link and its discontent

We can reconstruct this mythical foundation in the ontogenesis of the set by what couples explicitly say about their beginning. We can learn about an additional source of what brought them together by listening to their complaints and recriminations. The complaints express their disappointment about one another or the link and reveal the experience of a lost Paradise. We can presume, therefore, that they believe in the illusion of having had the same illusion – that there was a shared phantasy of the togetherness, which is now lost. Through their mutual recriminations, they unconsciously aspire to recover what has been lost, to erase the disappointment: "If this unpleasant situation weren't happening, we could go back to living in Paradise." Recriminations in the couple can be considered to be attempts to reinstate that mythical founding moment because they are suffering from the shattering of the initial illusion of falling in love. It is a moment of extreme susceptibility when the couple faces the possibility that Paradise is only a mirage. Another source of pain is added to this feeling of failure. When consensus collapses, words often operate mainly in their performative dimension. Their main function is not to transmit meaning, but to induce action: to convince, persuade, influence, or impose a way of being. The unconscious effort of the couple to recover the original and imaginary well-being of Paradise demands that a culprit for this loss be found. Additionally, unavoidable differences must be eliminated because they are experienced as shattering the fusional order that accounts for the couple's identificatory foundations.

Returning to John and Mary, the couple presented earlier in this paper, the reason they were coming to therapy can be understood as a story about what it means to attempt to go back to Paradise. They believed that conflicts do not belong in Paradise, and neither does miscommunication. The Paradise of the narcissistic foundational myth gave substance to their shared identity: in Paradise, couple members see everything in the same way. There is no conflict. They do not raise their voices. They do not argue or take offence to whatever the other says. The only conversations that are acceptable are "normal" and coherent.

Discontent resulting from disillusion, and from an inability to sustain a total togetherness, erases the sense of a "we" embodied in the representation of the set. More precisely, it deletes the idealised "we." Instead, the failed encounter feels like a catastrophic two-fold threat. On the one hand, there is the threat represented by the fact that the partner is not who he/she was. It is as if, suddenly, an unexpected other appears who is signified as a stranger and experienced as malicious, crazy, or uncanny. In fact, we should not see this experience as the emergence of a true stranger. When disillusion enters the stage, what emerges is the experience of an unexpected bewildering or persecuting other, but one who is not actually foreign. By experiencing the other as evil-minded, disrespecting, selfish, or absent, the otherness of the other can be eliminated, and they cease to be experienced as an unknown stranger. On the other hand, the dissolution of the idealised phantasy entails the threat of "not being us anymore" and unsettles the representation of the link itself. So, when the illusion of love is shattered, so is identity. The pain of the loss is compounded by a failure. Partners feel that something has, indeed, been lost and that they "are no longer what we used to be."

The ways in which the couple deals with this failure potentially give rise to different forms of violence that can result in polarisation (Aulagnier, 2001). When differences are seen as opposite versions, conflict can escalate. Partners might be able to discuss their differences, but they will be felt to be irresolvable when differences are experienced as contradictions. In the latter case, one version excludes, annihilates, or suppresses the other. The differences can even be ignored. It is as if the different idea, as well as the partner, does not exist. When this kind of polarisation is operating, the link itself is felt to be a threat to subjective identity, and each partner struggles to survive through the exertion of imposition and power.

## A short illustration

JOHN: I came back yesterday from a trip. We hardly saw each other this week. So, we didn't argue. Well … until last night.

MARY: I've been very busy these days. But you just came through the door and you're already complaining!

JOHN: I didn't complain. I arrived, I was hungry, you were not home; I called you to ask if I should wait for you to eat dinner. You said, no.

MARY: I didn't say that!

JOHN: You did say it.

MARY: I told you: Do what you want.

JOHN: It's the same thing.

MARY: It's not the same thing.

JOHN: After several days where we hadn't seen each other, I'd have expected you to say we would have dinner together.

MARY: I don't see why, since when I came back you gave me a dirty look. You always give me a look that stops me from wanting to do anything.

JOHN: It's not always like that; I'd have liked you to tell me to wait for you. But no. You let me eat on my own.

MARY: I also thought we'd eat together! But if you call and say you're hungry, how can I tell you to wait for me? You didn't even notice that I had prepared your favorite dessert!

In this short fragment we can see how painful it was for John and Mary to each learn that, unbeknownst to one another, they were both waiting for the other – that they both wanted to eat and be together. This is the moment where language collapsed, and John and Mary could not recognise the polysemy of words and gestures. Instead, they assumed that words have a univocal meaning. It seems as if John thought that he had phoned with the expectation that Mary would say she would have dinner with him. But it seems that Mary believed that just the fact that he asked about dinner meant he was hungry and wanted to eat immediately. Both the questions and the answers seem to have had different meanings for each of them. When Mary said, "Do what you want," John interpreted this to mean that she meant "No," while for Mary, it was a way of asking him to wait for her. They were annoyed by their disappointment that things did not work out as each had expected, and they were blaming each other for this failed encounter.

Their misunderstanding was the result of their taking for granted that they understood each other, while at the same time ignoring that words have different meanings according to each person's subjectivity. Their annoyance and recriminations concealed the disappointment that they couldn't find a way to understand each other. This lack of understanding was taken as evidence of disillusionment, which they believed should not be part of the link. Annoyance and recriminations emerged, each of them believing him or herself to be right and reasonable, blaming the other for the failed encounter. They both believed that it was because of the other's behaviour that they were not the couple they thought they were. They no longer looked at themselves in an idealised manner and felt that they were not the couple they once were. It is as if everything had collapsed.

This illustrates the unavoidable discrepancy between the individual internal representation of the couple and the couple created as a result of the other's presence. Reproaches, in this context, are both testimony to the dissolution of the representation of the link and, simultaneously, an attempt to recover it.

Let us imagine that after the analyst had interpreted along the line of some of the ideas discussed above and the session had continued.

JOHN: Oh, yes! We are so prickly, so sensitive!

MARY: Yes. It's understandable. It's a difficult time; we lose our temper easily.

JOHN: I will confess something to you. Last night I did see the rice pudding ... but I was so upset that the last thing I wanted was to eat it. But this morning I tried it. [Mary looks at him with a smile.] It was delicious.

MARY: Yesterday, when I realised that you hadn't even tried it, I was going to throw it out.

JOHN: Really? Would you have dared?

MARY: I was furious. I wanted to kill you. Did you really think I'd rather you ate alone?

JOHN: (looking at her tenderly) Yes!

It is remarkable how the climate of the encounter has changed. Now, both John and Mary can experience and name the new representation of their togetherness: being sensitive and prickly. When they describe themselves in this way, they find a new representation of the set. When they are able to find a name for it in an atmosphere that has ceased to be exasperating, both of them are feeling that they have suffered a misunderstanding. A new representation emerges: they can both look at it and feel they both belong to it. This new representation is a new "we." Now, differences are recognised and even tolerated. It is a state of radical difference (Kaës, 1989). Instead of recriminating each other, they start to be interested in thinking about "What happened to us?"; "How did we arrive at this point?"; and "How is it possible to be so misunderstood?"

Discontent is now finding its place as something inherent and intrinsic to the link, as being part of a set, a feeling that is now acceptable to John and Mary. When the other is experienced as somebody surprising, an unexpected stranger, rather than a negative and rejected known-other, there is an opportunity to see the other in his or her otherness, in their alienness.

The tenderness that can emerge in the couple under these conditions creates an atmosphere of intimacy. In this emotional state, the other can be regarded in his or her otherness, and one's own sense of identity will also be affected by the look of the other. If this emotional experience can be sustained for at least a short while, the alienness of the other can be contained instead of eliminated through persuasion or denial, and even curiosity and a desire to know that other may be aroused. A failed encounter can lead to a new encounter, one which we know will always be transient. This encountering in the failed encounter (Moguillansky and Seiguer, 1996) creates privileged and fleeting moments (or linking states of mind) that are always fluctuating.

When they participate in this depressive position climate, both members of the couple can recognise that it is the link itself – the fact of not being alone but with an other – that subjects them to the impossibility of full and immediate understanding. In other words, this could be considered a link version of castration. The inconsistency of the link can be recognised and accepted, and this allows a step forward towards a transformation of the persecutory enunciation – "You've done it to me" – to a depressive experience (Bion, 1965). Radical alienness can be contained thanks to confidence, which renders sincerity possible: "To say what you mean and to mean what you say," as Meltzer (1994) puts it.

During this emotional experience, the individual ego is again "decentered," so to speak, but there is no narcissistic offence. It is as though they could look at each other and say:

"You were horrible."

"You too. Anyway, I love you."

"Me too."

Confidence means supporting the hope for a new encounter after the failed encounter has occurred. This confidence has a generative capacity and requires that both partners be willing to be signified by the other, to lose something of their own identity, and to accept the way in which they are looked at or thought of by their partner, even if this way of looking or thinking does not coincide with their own.

## Final remarks

Couple psychodynamics can be viewed as an ongoing fluctuation between fusional emotional states underlying the identity of togetherness and moments of disillusionment where the other, as an other, is forced to fit into the narcissistic representation of the set. Complaints and recriminations provide a clinical compass to examine the unconscious meanings underlying such fluctuations.

Every emotional state is fragile and unstable, and couples always try to propose solutions aimed towards security, pictured as a changeless fusional being. To this end, they stress similarities, extol coincidences, and negate or disavow differences that do not contribute to the construction of a unity. The search for security crystallises in routines, customs, traditions, shared memories, and histories that must not be changed or questioned (Freud, 1899, 1912, 1930). While we know that security is a mirage, it produces the effect of an achievement and renews the illusion of a shared representation, creating a fictional stabilisation in a seamless "we." However, when the fear of dissolution is strong and cannot be contained, the need for an idealised "we" may lead the couple to cling to the security of traditions in a way that devitalises and impoverishes them, leaving no room for that which is new to enter the life of the couple.

In contrast, when the members of a couple are able to contain and work through the illusory narcissistic foundation of the link, and contain the disillusion without resorting to security, a new other and a new representation of the set can be welcomed as a novelty worthy of experience. It is within the state of the emotional link that the presence of the other, as an other, can be recognised as such.

# References

Aulagnier, P. (2001). *The violence of interpretation: From pictogram to statement.* London: Routledge.

Aulagnier, P. (2015). Birth of a body, origin of a history. *International Journal of Psychoanalysis*, 96(5), 1371.

Berenstein, I. (2001a). The link and the other. *International Journal of Psychoanalysis*, 82, 141–149.

Berenstein I. (2001b). El vínculo y el otro. *Revista de psicoanálisis de la APM* [*The Subject and the Other*], 35, 11–21.

Berenstein, I. (2012). Vínculo as a relationship between others. *Psychoanalytic Quarterly*, 81, 565–577.

Bion, W. (1965). *Transformations: Change from learning to growth.* London: Heinmann.

Freud, S. (1899). Screen memories. In J. Strachey (Ed. & Trans.), *The standard edition of the complete psychological works of Sigmund Freud* (Vol. 3, pp. 301–322). London: The Hogarth Press.

Freud, S. (1912). Remembering, repeating and working through. In *The standard edition of the complete psychological works of Sigmund Freud* (Vol. 12, pp. 147–156). London: The Hogarth Press.

Freud, S. (1914). On narcissism: An introduction. In *The standard edition of the complete psychological works of Sigmund Freud* (Vol. 14, pp. 67–100). London: The Hogarth Press.

Freud, S. (1930). Civilization and its discontents. *The standard edition of the complete psychological works of Sigmund Freud* (Vol. 21, pp. 57–146). London: The Hogarth Press.

Hobsbawm, E. & Ranger, T. (1983). *The invention of tradition.* Cambridge: Cambridge Press.

Kaës, R. (1989). El pacto denegativo en los conjuntos trans-subjetivos [The denegative pact in trans-subjective groups]. In: A. Missenard, J. Guillaumin, G. Rosolato, J. Kristeva, Y. Gutiérrez, J.-J. Baranes, R. Moury, R. Roussillon, & R. Kaës (Eds.), *Lo negativo. Figuras y modalidades* [*The negative: figures and modes*] (pp. 130–169). Buenos Aires: Amorrortu, 1991.

Meltzer, D. (1994). *Sincerity and other works* (pp. 185–284). London: Karnac Books. (Original work published 1971)

Moguillansky, R. & Seiguer, G. (1996). *La vida emocional de la familia.* [*The emotional life of the family English Translation?*]. Lugar: Buenos Aires.

# Chapter 14

# Discussion of "Approaching couples through the lens of Link Theory"

*Julie Friend*

I want to thank Monica Vorchheimer for bringing us this extremely rich and complex exposure to Link Theory in relation to the work of psychoanalytic couple psychotherapy. We are very fortunate. She has distilled a large body of theoretical literature that is complicated and new for most of us. We are treated to her focused perspective on Link Theory as it relates specifically to the complex world of psychoanalytic work with couples. She is highly qualified to lead us down this road, and the research is groundbreaking.

It is also a challenging chapter since there is so much new information to think about, and since Vorchheimer's thinking is layered, often moving in several directions simultaneously and endeavouring to communicate the complexity of the relationship between two psychoanalytic views of the human psyche, two lexicons, and two logics. In Puget's (2010) words, "The logic of the psychic world, which we have been unfolding and exploring in great depth since Freud, and the logic of the relational (linkage) world do not coincide" (pp. 5–6).

Vorchheimer's point of entry into the relationship between these two logics is her observation of something quite familiar to us: a couple's catastrophic reaction to a loss of understanding, which she enlists as a way of bringing together two avenues of psychoanalytic thought to bear on a third arena of focus – the couple relationship. On the one hand of this exploration, we have our familiar lineage and body of theory, resting on Freud's elucidation of the importance of internalisation, repetition, and internal representation in psychic life. On the other hand, there is the world of Link Theory and the exploration and highlighting of the ongoing importance of presentation, immediacy, and social structure. In her chapter, Vorchheimer is showing us how these two logics, these two lexicons, can be thought about in relation to psychoanalytic couple psychotherapy.

DOI: 10.4324/9781003265023-14

Link Theory not only challenges (or at least expands) some of our most basic operating assumptions, but it also importantly adds a social, cultural, and perhaps a political perspective that is too commonly lacking, or ancillary, in psychoanalytic theory. Before I attempt to highlight more carefully some of the central ideas that Vorchheimer is proposing in her chapter, I would like to see if I can get some sense of what is different about Link Theory.

Central to Link Theory, in contrast to the psychoanalysis we are most familiar with, is the recognition of the impact of the presence of a unique subject—in addition to an internal representation – on our experience and our psychic life. For example, Vorchheimer comes from another country, from another culture, with a different way of thinking, of speaking, and using different points of reference. She lives in relation to different cultural and social links, and they are part of her uniqueness. What has it been like to read her paper? Maybe you are excited by these ideas; maybe also puzzled. How do the challenges of confusion, uncertainty, excitement, and lack of familiarity impact you? Did you find yourself looking for similarities or familiarities in what Vorchheimer was saying, things you could feel you "know"?

The ideas Vorchheimer brings are new to most of us. According to Link Theory, her alterity inherently disrupts – and disturbs – our familiar ways of thinking about our work, our links with our own professional history – our teachers, our analysts, and maybe our sense of place in the community. How do you experience her presence and the presentation of her ideas and thinking? How possible is it to remain curious, to tolerate being uncertain, intrigued, or confused? Do you find yourself spacing out, or perhaps notice a need to overwrite the newness, the disturbance inherent in this encounter, with a sense of quick understanding, or of dismissiveness, or of idealisation? What is it like to encounter a new, unique person in the present moment?

It may be useful, too, in making sense of Vorchheimer's contribution, to consider the context in which Link Theory was developed, first by Pichon-Riviere, and later developed by the Berensteins, Puget, Bleger, and others, in Argentina in the 1960s and 1970s. It is not coincidental that this very period of time was extremely disturbing and tumultuous in much of Latin America. In Argentina, The Process of National Reorganization, also known as "The Dirty War," was the name used for a violent and terrorising campaign by the Argentine government against anyone they viewed as dissidents.

During this time, military and government security forces systematically hunted down, tortured, and killed anyone believed to be associated with socialism or Marxism. This included labour union members, artists, intellectuals, university students and professors, clergy, and psychoanalysts. The official estimates of the number dead or disappeared – people who were never found, dead or alive – is generally stated as between 13,000 and 30,000 and, in fact, may be much higher.

In an atmosphere of such social terror and turmoil, it would be unthinkable to consider our world, and our experience of it, as principally an outcome of our unconscious or infantile experience, of representation and repetition alone. Link Theory describes a wider concept than that of an object relationship and always includes the unalterable impact of the alterity of the other and of the external world on our psychic life. Link Theory makes a place to think about the ongoing "dialectical interrelation of the external and internal worlds" (Bernardi and De Leon De Bernardi, 2012, p. 537).

Vorchheimer's evocative descriptions aid our understanding of this theoretical realm. She tells us Link Theory makes a place for us to think about "the inscriptions arising within the fabric of human relations." Her choice of the word "inscription," and later also of the word "stamp," is instructive: both words describe a defining impact from outside of something onto its surface. Both words suggest some force and pressure. "Inscribe" implies the scraping of a surface to leave a mark, an image that perhaps implies some breaking of a boundary. Both actions leave an indelible impression that changes, defines, names, or claims something. This is a wonderful way, I think, of communicating that every encounter can change us and impact our experience, our identity, our place of belonging, our way of thinking. We are indelibly and unavoidably impacted by external reality and by the fact that we are "in a web of significant others" who have an ongoing effect on us. This idea emphasizes that the psychic apparatus is open to new inscriptions and not only re-inscriptions of memory traces. I find this a hopeful and refreshing perspective.

Link Theory makes a place for thinking theoretically about the impact of *an other*, whose "alterity is irreducible" (Berenstein, 2001, p. 144). In Vorchheimer's words, we are "moulded not only by the relationship to the body ego and the drives but also by the link with the other and with the social background" (this volume, p. 167).

Links also cohere the social fabric, and I will say more about that shortly. In these terms, every interaction is embedded in and represents a structure we are part of, contributes to our place in the social structure, and, simultaneously, every new interaction is potentially disruptive, perhaps inherently so, and as such represents a demand for a new adjustment, for psychic work. This adjustment is at once intrapsychic, social, and relational. Centrally, we are not isolates. And, implicitly, the possibilities for development and change are ongoing, if we can bear the disturbance of the encounter with each other in a creative way, a way that doesn't occlude difference.

Onto the matrix of the complexity of Link Theory, Vorchheimer opens the equally complex world of couple relationships. We know from our work with couples that alterity can be a tall order indeed. The pull towards accord, alignment, and agreement in couples can be gravitational and, as Vorchheimer illustrates through the case of John and Mary, a lack of understanding can be experienced as destructive, catastrophic, murderous, and hateful – the list can go on. We have all witnessed plenty of these moments, I am sure.

We are familiar with thinking about these sorts of couple interactions in terms of narcissistic relating, as has been described by James Fisher and Stan Ruszczynski, in both their numerous publications. From our familiar intrapsychic, representational perspective, for example, Fisher (1999) tells us that narcissism is:

> [...] a kind of object relating in which there is an intolerance for the reality, the independent existence of the other. Narcissism in this sense is, in fact, a longing for an other, but a longing for an other who is perfectly attuned and responsive, and thus not a genuine other at all.
>
> (pp. 1–2)

Here, narcissism is viewed through the lens of object relations, with implicitly historical roots, highlighting the role of projection of internal objects onto one's partner. Those of us working in this way are familiar with watching for the ways in which couples construct their relationship via projection and projective identification, frequently obstructing the reality of each other, and we know something from observing their internal object worlds play out before our eyes. We are accustomed to thinking of narcissistic difficulties in intrapsychic, developmental terms and directing our interventions accordingly.

Bringing in Link Theory, Vorchheimer extends our understanding of narcissism in couples. She describes how a couple exceeds the personal, and how the fact of being in a couple redefines them as a set, a unit of social structure. A couple also creates a new social order, one that implicitly replaces – Loewald (1979) might say, "murders" – the old. A couple, therefore, is not only an important personal structure and experience but is also a part of the social structure and represents a new identity, a new social set, a new order, and a sense of "non-fleeting existence" in the minds of the couple and in their community. This is a very important idea that adds depth to our understanding of the desperation couples can feel when they experience their partner as too different from the partner they think they know.

In what I think is a brilliant turn in her paper, Vorchheimer brings Freud back into the picture. In so doing, she enhances and clarifies our understanding of the link and its importance for our understanding of couples. She says narcissism in couples can be seen to represent a particular kind of ubiquitous, human link, and constitutes a "foundational myth." Through that lens, she reminds us of the ways in which a baby is invested by her parents with carrying hope for the future, and identities from the past, investments that link the child with the social contract and contribute to a sense of coherent identity, for both individuals and their communities. Vorchheimer's unique contribution in this paper is to extend this idea to couples: she tells us that a couple, too, is invested with a foundational myth, and this provides a sense of a secure, solid, unitary identity. This myth, she notes, is fundamentally narcissistic in nature, and, because of this, it tends to turn the partners away from the inevitability of difference. With this important contribution, Vorchheimer enables us to think of a couple relationship in new ways: it is not only a relationship between two people, each with their own internal object world, each with their own different history and social links. But also, she reminds us, a couple represents a new social order, a social contract, and structure, as well. At the same time, she reminds us that we cannot forget that a couple is not solid or immutable, as people in a relationship would like very much to believe: a couple is an emotional experience, fed by phantasy, always in flux.

Vorchheimer emphasises that since the formation of a couple is in part based on an experience of reconstituting paradise and infantile narcissism, of perfection and limitless possibility, misunderstanding or the loss of understanding is experienced as a catastrophic destruction or erasure of paradise. Implicit in this dense idea is the attribution by the community of a perfect and idealised couple onto the couple, similar to parents attributing perfection to their infant.

Vorchheimer's contribution helps us better understand the importance of the link and the representation of the set in couples' minds. To underscore this, she once again uses an evocative, illuminating word. She tells us that within the illusion of love that captivates and defines a newly formed couple, "a sense of perfection overflies couples when in love, concealing defects." "Overflies" – a wonderful word – it evokes soaring, defying gravity, over-reaching ... maybe transgressing ... and brings to mind, for me, Chagall's images of lovers rising, entwined, above the rooftops in the night. It is an image that embodies both the exaltation and the unreality of the narcissism embedded in the couple link. When one overflies, there is the inevitable crash to earth, like the bitter, angry moments Vorchheimer tells us about between Mary and John.

In highlighting this element of a couple link, I think Vorchheimer adds a valuable and unique perspective on narcissism for us. She highlights how a loss of understanding is a threat not only for the reasons we have been familiar with – the intolerance of difference, the need for omnipotent control, the need for the partner to receive and contain certain projections, or the longing for a particular quality of relationship to repair past traumas. Misunderstanding or not understanding also challenges a vision of perfection that underpins a couple identity. Difference can threaten their sense of identity as a couple, an identity that links the couple together, secures a sense of identity, and also links them to the fabric of social life. Vorchheimer says this experience "could be considered a linkage version of castration" (this volume, p. 177). In this light, the flaw or imperfection represented by misunderstanding is easier to understand as constituting an unbearable threat and catastrophe.

If we accept that identity as a couple is underpinned by a narcissistic myth, then when difference emerges, as it does in these moments of not understanding between Mary and John, we can more fully understand the magnitude of the impact this difference could represent to them. In Vorchheimer's view, it is because the difficulty in understanding and the differences between them mean that, since they are no longer perfect, they are no longer a set; they are no longer who they were and can no longer can rely on their identity as a set and on their place in the social order. She thus helps us understand the catastrophic quality of betrayal that can sometimes accompany moments of lack of understanding between people in couple relationships.

But, we know difference is inevitable. What enables some couples, sometimes, to manage difference, manage the injury difference represents from this perspective? How does the addition of Link Theory to our thinking affect our clinical choices? What are we aiming to help the couple face and develop, and how do we do this?

Vorchheimer's viewpoint is represented by her view that: there is an unavoidable discrepancy between the individual internal representation of the couple and the couple which is created as a result of the presence of the other. Somehow this fact, this reality, must come to be made part of the structure of the link between the couple, which otherwise has only an inherently narcissistic basis. I think she suggests that we must help them face the loss of an ideal, in this case, the loss of a fantasy of perfection that overflies reality.

I think she is telling us that in order to accept this more limited reality, the narcissistic vision and hope embodied in the link binding the couple must be recognised and mourned, like any experience of castration. If this can be made possible, the couple can better face disjunctures, misunderstandings, and differences with some curiosity and tenderness. To put it another way, there must be an expansion of their idea of coupling, to include inevitable imperfection and discontent. She states that difference is more manageable for couples if "Each member of the link must make, produce, a space for the otherness in the relationship" (Berenstein, 2009, p. 1).

So, how do we, as couple psychotherapists, do this? Let's go back to the interchange between John and Mary. We meet them at a moment of reunion following a separation and hear about their hurtful misunderstanding of one another (this volume, pp. 174–175 volume):

JOHN: *I didn't complain; I arrived, I was hungry, you were not at home.*
  *I phoned asking if I should wait for you for dinner. You said: no.*
MARY: *I didn't say that!*

And later:

JOHN: *It's not always like that; I'd have liked you to tell me to wait for*
  *you. But no. You left me eating alone.*

MARY: *I also thought we'd eat together! But if you call saying you are hungry, how was I going to tell you to wait for me? You didn't even notice that I had prepared your favourite dessert!*

It is interesting to consider how Vorchheimer might approach such moments in the consulting room. I am curious to know how she *does* intervene, and what she might say, particularly because Link Theory describes such an important, ubiquitously human, dilemma. How would her approach differ from our more familiar, representational perspective, in which we might wonder: what do separations mean to each of them; how needs are managed by this couple and what do they signify; how would we understand that neither says, "Hello", or "Welcome home, I missed you," or "It was great having time to myself," or "Shall we eat dinner together?"

Vorchheimer mentions the importance of the idea of "confidence" in her approach to helping couples, which she says helps the partners [build] a disposition to be signified by the other, to lose something of one's own identity, to accept the way in which [they] are looked at or thought of by our partner, even if this does not coincide with our own viewpoint.

I have been wondering what she means by confidence and have come to think she may be pointing towards the importance of offering an experience of containment to the couple. Vorchheimer's ideas on Link Theory allow us an expanded understanding of the impact of misunderstandings. To our familiar thinking about the unique, developmental elements in each member of the couple that colour their particular experiences of misunderstanding, she compellingly adds the consequential, universal dilemma that the couple is facing in such moments, too. I think an important implication of Vorchheimer's idea is that, with this broadened appreciation of the impact that misunderstanding can have on the couple, we may be more able to communicate our understanding of the layered magnitude of their particular distress, and, as Bion (1959) says, "retain a balanced outlook" when there is an experience of not understanding each other. This increased understanding enables us to offer a fuller experience of containment, one that could help the couple metabolise and bear more of their experience, mourn and develop, and better bear the truth of one another.

Vorchheimer's rich, layered, groundbreaking paper offers an enormous amount to think about. To our existing corpus of psychoanalytic theory about couples, she adds Link Theory, a perspective that broadens – and destabilises – our existing framework. Her paper, like an encounter with an other, creates a demand for work on our part in order to understand and incorporate a novel perspective. It shifts our centre of gravity. She helps us see that a couple is many things: a link, a social contract, a dream of a perfect future, a return to paradise, a fantasy, and an ever-shifting emotional experience.

As any excellent, innovative paper does, Vorchheimer's contribution raises more questions than it answers: How does Link Theory translate in the consulting room? How can we marry Link Theory with developmental thinking? We know that psychic capacity has an impact on the couple's ability to struggle with and manage misunderstandings and differences. How might we map what sorts of couple relationships struggle more, or less, with the inherent unpredictability of relating to one another, and struggle more with the universal, human dilemma she is elucidating?

Certainly, Vorchheimer brings to our attention the necessity for us, as couple psychotherapists, to strengthen our own capacity to bear and hold a space for a broad, destabilised view of couple connection and couple life. I think she points us towards the importance of our capacity to tolerate the confusion, disjunctures, and shifts that are ubiquitous in any relationship.

I want to thank Vorchheimer for this excellent paper, for her scholarly and creative theoretical connections, for the important reminder to include the impact of social reality in our thinking, and for her evocative language. The addition of Link Theory to our psychoanalytic corpus reminds us to stay aware of the ubiquitous and inevitable pull couples can experience in order to escape awareness of the fragility and instability of connection, and of their effort to generate 'solutions' in order to secure a sense of similarity, fusion, and an illusion of a shared representation.

## References

Berenstein, I. (2001). The link and the other. *International Journal of Psychoanalysis*, *82*, 141–149.

Berenstein, I. (2009). The concept of the link in couple and family psychoanalysis. Part 1. *International Review of Psychoanalysis of Couple and Family*, *6*(2), 1–3.

Bernardi, R. & De Leon De Bernardi, B. (2012). The concepts of *vínculo* and dialectical spiral: A bridge between intra- and intersubjectivity. *Psychoanalytic Quarterly*, *81*, 531–564.

Bion, W.R. (1959). Attacks on linking. *International Journal of Psycho-Analysis, 40*, 308–315.

Fisher, J.V. (1999). *The uninvited guest*. London: Karnac Books.

Loewald, H.W. (1979). The waning of the Oedipus complex. *Journal of the American Psychoanalytic Association, 27*, 751–775.

Puget, J. (2010). The subjectivity of certainty and the subjectivity of uncertainty. *Psychoanalytic Dialogues, 20*, 4–20.

## Chapter 15

# The application of contemporary Self Psychology to couple psychotherapy

*Carla Leone*

## Introduction

> Throughout his life a person will experience himself as a cohe-sive harmonious firm unit in time and space, connected with his past and pointing meaningfully into a creative-productive future, only as long as, at each stage of his life, he experiences certain representatives of his human surrounding as joyfully responding to him, as available to him as sources of idealized strength and calmness, as being silently present but in essence like him, and, at any rate, able to grasp his inner life more or less accurately so that their responses are attuned to his needs and allow him to grasp their inner life when he is in need of such sustenance.
>
> (Kohut, 1984, pp. 51–52)

This description of what people need from each other and their envi-ronment resonated with me and piqued my interest in Self Psychology from the minute I read it. I immediately thought of its implications for couple and family therapy, as it seemed to beautifully capture the kinds of experiences partners and family members need from each other – and from their therapists. The more I learned about Self Psychology – through reading Kohut's original work and that of many who came after him – the more helpful I found it in my work with couples and families, as well as individual patients. This chapter summarises my view of the theory's major contributions to work with couples, includ-ing my belief that psycho-educational or advice-giving interventions can be consistent with its basic tenets in many cases.

A growing literature has discussed the application of Self Psychology to the treatment of couples, beginning in the late 1980s (Leone, 2008,

DOI: 10.4324/9781003265023-15

2013a, 2018, 2019; Livingston, 1995, 1998, 2001a, 2001b, 2007; Ringstrom, 1994; Shaddock, 1998, 2000; Solomon, 1988; Trop, 1994, 1997). Most of these authors also incorporated concepts from the intersubjective systems theory proposed by Stolorow and his colleagues (see, for example, Stolorow, Brandshaft & Atwood, 1987), and Ringstrom (2012, 2014, 2018) recently integrated both of these with concepts from American Relational theory (see, for example, Mitchell & Aron, 1999). A few authors have noted that there is often an educating component to psychoanalytic couple treatment (Livingston, 2001b; MacIntosh, 2019) and/ or have presented cases in which some educating-type responses were included (see, for example, Pizer & Pizer, 2006). I have been influenced by all of this work and intend this chapter to build on and extend it.

## Understanding couples and their difficulties

The tenets of Self Psychology I see as most relevant to understanding couples include:-

- The concept of selfobject experience and selfobject needs.
- The idea that even overtly very dysfunctional behaviour can have a "forward edge" or "leading edge."
- Viewing the sense of self as central to health and functioning, including relational functioning.

I will discuss each briefly before moving to treatment principles and their application to couple therapy.

*Selfobject experience and needs:* Kohut defined selfobject experience somewhat differently at different times, but the quote I opened with best illustrates the way I use it: selfobject experience is a dimension of our experience of others or the environment that functions to strengthen our sense of self and sense of connection. This includes any experience that is affirming, vitalising, comforting, or otherwise enhancing; one that increases the felt sense of being understood, resonated with, and responded to in an attuned manner. Kohut proposed three types of selfobject experience: mirroring; idealising; and twinship experience and posited that we need all three throughout life for healthy development and functioning (Kohut, 1984). Later authors suggested that all three can be seen as different ways to help process affect (Stolorow, Brandshaft & Atwood, 1987).

Although Kohut never discussed the potential application of his work to couple therapy, in the end notes of his last book he commented on "the mutual selfobject functions that partners in a good marriage provide for each other" (Kohut, 1984, p. 220). He also repeated his frequent quip that "a good marriage is one in which only one partner is crazy at a time" (Kohut, 1984, p. 220), and explained this means "a good marriage is one in which one or the other partner rises to the challenge of providing the selfobject functions that the other's temporarily impaired self needs at a particular moment" (Kohut, 1984, p. 220). Thus, healthy couples can be seen as functioning as a reliable source of selfobject experience for each other, in a mutual, reciprocal, "good-enough" (Winnicott, 1953) manner. Kohut's emphasis on the rupture and repair process between analyst and patient (see, for example, Kohut, 1984), discussed below, suggests that well-functioning couples are also able to process inevitable empathic ruptures well and repair their connection fairly quickly. This is consistent with findings of later empirical studies (Gottman, 1999).

Troubled, conflictual, or disengaged couples are not able to reliably function this way, for a number of reasons. From this perspective, all couples' difficulties stem from a lack of needed selfobject experience, or selfobject failures between the partners. These failures can be due to partners having conflicting or opposite selfobject needs simultaneously, as when saving money is a selfobject experience for one, but spending promotes selfobject experience for the other. They can also be due to partners lacking the abilities or capacities needed to function adequately as a source of selfobject experience for another, including the abilities to:

- identify and express their own feelings and needs.
- listen for, understand, and respond in an attuned manner to the other's subjective experience and needs.
- tolerate some disappointment when their needs are not met.
- compromise, negotiate, and apologise effectively.

These abilities are, in turn, influenced by the extent to which individuals have developed:

- a positive, cohesive sense of self.
- the ability to experience, regulate, and integrate affect effectively.

- the ability to mentalise, or reflect on one's own experience and the imagined (different) experience of the other (see, for example, Fonagy & Target, 1997; Fonagy et al., 2004).
- organising principles about the self, others, relationships, and the world (Stolorow, Brandshaft & Atwood, 1987) and implicit or procedural relational knowledge (see, for example, Lyons-Ruth et al., 1998; Lyons-Ruth,1999) that support or promote attuned selfobject responsiveness.

Relationships are also influenced by the patterns of interaction that emerge between partners over time, such as pursue-distance, attack-defend, and so on. Couple treatment needs to target any and all of these factors when they interfere with reliable selfobject experience between the partners.

*The "forward edge" of problematic behaviour*: The forward edge refers to the healthy, growth-seeking aspects of otherwise dysfunctional behaviour – or "what the patient is trying to attain, retain, or maintain" (Lachmann, 2016, p. 501) through the behaviour, such as bolstering a vulnerable sense of self, retaining an attachment, or regulating states of over- or under-stimulation (Lachmann, 2016). Since partners in couple therapy frequently present with markedly problematic behaviour, this is an especially useful concept for couple therapists.

Kohut did not write much about this concept himself, but referred to the idea in consultation with supervisees (Miller, 1985; see also Sandmeyer, 2019; Tolpin, 2002). In addition to having a leading or forward edge, problematic behaviours are also seen as having a "trailing edge," a more traditional psychoanalytic concept referring to the behaviour's painful origins or what the patient is repeating or defending against.

Two problematic behaviours commonly seen in couple therapy – contempt and defensiveness – can be understood as having both trailing and leading edges. Both can be seen as efforts to defend against or avoid painful feelings of inadequacy – the behaviour's "trailing edge," or, as attempts to bolster or preserve a fragile or shaky sense of self (by positioning oneself as superior), its forward edge. Contempt and other forms of aggression can also be a way to protest or try to stop perceived hurtful or threatening behaviour and/or to communicate (by impact) the experience of shame or distress, both forward edge efforts. Framing problematic behaviour as motivated in part by a healthy need or goal often feels accurate and validating for patients and makes it easier for them to acknowledge the behaviour's trailing edge or problematic aspects. "Some degree of defensiveness is natural and understandable," I often tell couples, and remind them that people need to feel safe and well-connected to be able to drop their protective defences and examine themselves self-critically.

*The centrality of the sense of self:* Kohut believed that a positive, cohesive sense of self was central to psychological health and adaptive functioning, and that a shaky or negative sense of self underlies most pathology or difficulties, presumably including relationship difficulties. Given the mutual narcissistic injuries partners so often cause each other, this concept is particularly useful in understanding couples and their behaviour, such as intense reactions to seemingly minor slights. Viewing the sense of self as central and crucial suggests that couple therapists should monitor the state of the self of each partner closely and help them learn to do so with each other.

## Treatment principles and methods

*Goal of treatment:* From this perspective, the overall goal of couple therapy is to improve partners' abilities to function as a reliable source of selfobject experience for each other. For some couples, this can involve just a little fine-tuning or help repairing a rupture and resuming the well-functioning selfobject relationship they previously had. But for many others, including those with a history of trauma and/or early, pervasive selfobject failure, it can involve a much longer, complex process of learning selfobject relating or functioning from scratch, including gradually developing the capacities and abilities listed above. And of course, most couples fall somewhere in between. Couple therapy can look extremely different depending on the extent to which partners have already acquired these capacities – or not.

*Theory of change:* Kohut's work is consistent with the view later espoused by the Boston Process of Change Group (see, for example, Boston Change Process Study Group, 2008) and others (Fosshage, 2005; Herzog, 2011) that change occurs through two overlapping pathways: (1) new ideas, insights, awarenesses, or ways of thinking, and (2) positive new, corrective relational experience. Although Kohut initially saw interpretation leading to insight as the primary mechanism of cure, he wrote extensively on the selfobject bond between analyst and patient, and shortly before his death acknowledged that empathy and the therapeutic relationship were therapeutic in themselves as well (Kohut, 1984). The two processes are not as separate as they might seem, since a new idea or insight arrived at in the presence of another or in collaboration with another can constitute a new relational experience, and new relational experiences can promote or lead to new insights or awarenesses.

*Treatment approach:* Toward these goals, specific treatment methods include:

- *Equal empathic immersion* into each partner's subjective affective experience: Kohut was concerned that many aspects of the classical approach took the analyst too far away from the patient's subjective affective experience. His writings on empathic immersion, vicarious introspection into the patient's inner world, listening from within the patient's subjective perspective or vantage point, and understanding first and explaining second (Kohut, 1959, 1971, 1977, 1981, 1984), are a widely recognised, perhaps revolutionary contribution to psychoanalysis. Yet as important as feeling deeply known and understood can be in individual treatment, it is perhaps even more crucial in couple therapy, where partners are so vulnerable and typically feel so deeply misunderstood by the very person they most love and need, or once loved and needed. For some partners, feeling deeply understood or "gotten" by the same person (their couple therapist) may be the first thing they have agreed on or had in common in years.

So, in every session, my goal first and foremost is for each partner to feel deeply understood and empathically responded to by me – before I worry about trying to help them see or do things differently. I especially strive for what I call "bullseyes" – moments when the therapist captures the patient's experience (in words, imagery, metaphor, tone, etc.) so closely that the patient says something like "Exactly!" or "Yes, that's it!" I usually settle for a nod, moment of assenting eye contact or even a shrug that says, "close enough," but I'm always trying for those bullseyes.

Being equally immersed in each partner's subjective experience, viewpoint and inner world is easier said than done, since it is natural for the couple therapist to understand or identify with one partner more easily than the other. However, it is crucial that the therapist monitor herself for this tendency and re-double her efforts to better understand the less-well-understood partner, as will be illustrated in the case example below.

- *Balanced attuned responsiveness and connectedness:* The therapist also attempts to function as a potential source of selfobject experience and connection for both partners as equally as possible. Bacal has discussed the therapist's "optimal responsiveness" (Bacal, 1985, 1998), in which the therapist uses her ever-deepening impression of each partner's inner world and emotional needs to make an educated guess as to the response that might be most strengthening or attuned to the patient's needs at any given moment. An empathic summary of the patient's subjective emotional experience that helps them feel deeply understood and known? A new idea (including an interpretation) or piece of information they hadn't thought of or known, and which might pique their interest, feel calming, or offer hope? Responses that highlight their strengths or normalise their struggles, which might feel affirming and reassuring? The therapist makes her best guess based on her multiply influenced intuition in the improvisational clinical moment (Stern, 2017), then watches closely to see how the response is received and adapts accordingly. This could involve repairing empathic ruptures if she was very far off, and always involves an ongoing process of trial and error, learning and adjustment leading to ever-greater attunement and patient-therapist "fittedness" (Sander, 1991; Stern, 2017) over time. The therapist strives for a relationship in which therapist and patient are a "felt presence" in each other's lives and feel a sense of connectedness, as described by Geist (2008, 2009, 2010, 2011, 2013, 2016).
- *Explaining or making sense together*: As with all psychoanalytic models, Self Psychology-informed couple treatment involves creating a safe space and fostering dialogue that promotes exploration and reflection, especially into each partner's more vulnerable or less accessible affective experience, through which new awarenesses, insights, perspectives, and understandings can emerge. This includes exploring partners' early and later experiences, their current relationship and its history, and the relationship between each partner and the therapist. However, in the Self Psychological

approach, the interpretive process is seen first and foremost as having a selfobject function – strengthening the sense of self and sense of connection – which is as important or therapeutic as the content or accuracy of the interpretation. All psychoanalytic approaches advocate timing interpretations thoughtfully, but Self Psychology is more specific in its view of the interpretive process as a selfobject function or experience (Geist, 2020; Herzog, 2011). The Self Psychologist's interpretive comments reflect the concepts outlined above: a focus on the patient's subjective affective experience, sense of self, preconscious organising principles, and implicit relational knowledge; the forward edge of behaviours, and the relational or systemic patterns that have developed between the partners.

- *Close attention to narcissistic vulnerability, narcissistic injury, and the rupture and repair sequence:* In addition to his emphasis on the sense of self, Kohut wrote extensively on the inevitable empathic ruptures that occur between patient and analyst and the curative aspects of processing and repairing them when they occur. This process is perhaps even more relevant in couple therapy, where empathic ruptures and misattunements occur even more frequently than they do in individual treatments. This is partly because the couple therapist has more to attend to, and is therefore more likely to miss something, and partly because injuries, misattunements, and selfobject failures between the partners are so frequent.

It is therefore crucial that the couple therapist closely track or monitor each partner's moment-to-moment sense of narcissistic injury or vulnerability – the state of the self of each – and move quickly to address empathic failures or ruptures and repair them. This should take precedence over other important work since nothing else productive is likely to happen if someone is feeling injured or threatened. The repair process involves clarifying the injured person's feelings and perceptions, and responding with understanding, validation and apologies when indicated (including by the therapist). Apologies by the therapist should not occur so quickly that patients feel pushed to forgive or let go of their anger too quickly, but also not so slowly that they feel the therapist is avoiding or delaying taking responsibility (Weiss, 2018).

- *Coaching, educating, advice-giving, etc*: With few exceptions (as noted above), psychoanalytic couple therapists don't talk much about coaching, educating, or advice-giving, although I think most do some of it. These kinds of directive interventions might still be met in some psychoanalytic circles with the classic response "that's not psychoanalytic" – and when they are the only or primary interventions I would agree, as I have discussed elsewhere (see, for example, Leone & MacIntosh, 2013). Yet, I have found there are many times when educating or advice-giving is the most empathically attuned response to a partner or to the couple's primary need of the moment, and best furthers the goals of a psychoanalytic couple therapy.

In the role of teacher/advisor, the couple therapist can be a source of idealising selfobject experience (Kohut, 1984) for the couple, in which the therapist is experienced as a source of guidance, wisdom, and support. As long as the therapist carefully considers the multiple possible reasons why a teacher-student or advisor-advisee configuration might be emerging in the transference-countertransference field at a given time, the judicious use of such interventions can be a useful part of a fundamentally psychoanalytic treatment. For example, an empathically attuned response from one partner – especially when it is a "bullseye" – can be a powerful, potentially healing moment, even if the response was facilitated, nudged, or even directed by the couple therapist. Over time, such moments can lead to healing and deepening connection between the partners, and eventually to their ability to have them without the therapist's psychoanalytically informed nudges or advice.

## Case example

My first session with Will and Andrea illustrates many of the concepts described above. This description is true to the spirit of what occurred as I recall it, but the material has been appropriately disguised and is, in some parts, an amalgam of two very similar cases.

Will and Andrea had recently moved to the Chicago area from the southwest, where both were from, due to a job promotion for Will. They had been married for seventeen years, during which they had chronically struggled with Will's complaints about Andrea's temper outbursts. Both were seriously considering divorce.

Will begins by explaining that he has come only reluctantly, mainly to describe the problem for me, but not necessarily to participate in the treatment of it. He explains that he and Andrea have a good relationship and a good life in many ways: two great kids, a nice house, and fun vacations as a family. Their only real problem is Andi's "anger management" problem. "I know this isn't politically correct to say in 'family systems theory' or whatever you therapists call it," he says,

> but it is the truth: she really is at least ninety per cent of the problem. And I really resent being back in yet another couple therapist's office when, in our case, it's really not an equally caused problem, it's really her problem.

Andrea rolls her eyes and sighs in exasperation. I can tell she's heard this all before, probably ad nauseum. I meet her eyes and, through "eye dialogue," shoot her a glance that I hope conveys that I recognise how Will's statement must have felt and that I know she will have a very different take, then return to meeting Will's eyes. I feel like we are sizing each other up. I experience him as condescending and off-putting, but also begin to see deep pain in his eyes and sense a desperate wish for someone to hear him, believe him, and take his truth seriously. I also feel slightly impressed with his boldness and bluntness and resonate a bit, for both personal and professional reasons, with what I see as a legitimate objection to the idea that every couple problem is always mutually caused.

I realise I already feel more sympathetic to Andrea than Will, and Andrea hasn't opened her mouth yet. So I quickly try to rebalance before answering – by intentionally trying harder to see things through Will's eyes or imagine being him. I try to imagine feeling that my marriage and life would be great if it wasn't for this one terrible thing my husband did that I had no control over. And that therapist after therapist had told me that this was a co-created problem that I was contributing to equally and refused to believe me that it was really only him. In a flash I can picture it and feel it with him and I'm back to a place of more equal empathic immersion.

So I nod and shrug and say something like, "Mmhmm, I get it: it's her anger, not yours, and she's the one expressing it badly, so she should deal with changing it, not you or the two of you. Is that it?" (I again make connecting eye contact with Andrea to convey that I haven't forgotten her, that I know she sees it differently and will hear her out in a minute.)

Will's eyes meet mine in surprise, a little taken aback. "Um ... yes," he says, "that's it exactly, thank-you." I feel relieved by this apparent bullseye and like I may have passed my first test. Will adds that of course he would be willing to try to help Andrea, or be supportive of her efforts, as long as she takes full responsibility for herself and her own behaviour. But that's not what happens; instead Andrea makes excuses for her outbursts or "meltdowns" – which have at times included screaming, slamming doors, and threatening divorce in front of their sons.

Outraged, Andrea interrupts to say that she only mentioned divorce in front of the boys once and had apologised to them and reassured them immediately, and that these outbursts only happen very rarely under extreme duress. Will scoffs at what he sees as yet another example of Andrea minimising and notes that by "extreme duress" she means things like PMS (pre-menstrual syndrome), stress, lack of sleep, or, mostly, something he, Will, has done or not done, as though that justifies her behaviour!

Nodding at him and shooting Andrea another "I'm coming to you in a minute" look, I say that, of course, no one wants their spouse to make excuses for behaviour that is really hurtful to them or, especially, their children. That we all need to feel the person we've chosen to spend our lives with and depend on is able to look at themselves honestly and non-defensively, admit their problems or growing edges, and commit to changing them. (Will, again pleasantly surprised, interrupts to agree emphatically, saying that if Andrea would only do that, everything would be fine.) I nod but signal that I wasn't finished and add that I think most people also want to feel the person they fell in love with and have chosen to grow old with really understands them and gets them, even when they are emotionally flooded and behaving badly, or at least wants to and tries to. Now Andrea's nodding emphatically and looking relieved, but Will looks wary. I catch his eye and say that understanding is not the same as excusing hurtful behaviour, and this seems to mollify him a little.

In a slightly calmer tone, Andrea says she is not trying to excuse her behaviour, she agrees that it's important to admit your problems and take responsibility for poor behaviour. She admits to having a temper at times, when she's very upset or provoked, but says she's working on it and has improved a lot. The problem isn't that she doesn't (using air quotes) "own" her problems, as Will puts it, it's that Will thinks he "owns his stuff," when he really doesn't. Will rolls his eyes and sighs in exasperation, but she ignores this and launches into an example of a time she came home exhausted after a long day, when Will and the boys had been home for hours, to find the house a complete disaster, backpacks dropped right in the doorway where they could be tripped over, laundry all over the floor only half done when Will had agreed to do it, and dinner not even started even though she left a note right on the fridge with instructions. Yes, she says, in those situations she's responsible for her own behaviour, but she doesn't think it's "making excuses" to feel entitled to be pretty upset! (Meanwhile, I am flashing on some extremely similar scenes I've walked into myself. I again note my easy resonance with Andrea's experience and caution myself to be careful to stay equally connected to Will's.)

In a patient, long-suffering tone, Will refutes Andrea's portrayal point by point, after noting that he's explained this to her multiple times already. That having a right to be upset doesn't mean a right to yell and "pitch a fit." That she is more than welcome to give him any feedback she wants to or needs to, as long as she says it nicely and kindly. "Is that really too much to ask of a grown woman?" he asks. Outraged, Andrea points to this as yet another example of Will's condescension and patronising attitude. Of course, she should try to speak nicely in most cases, she agrees, but Will makes no room whatsoever for even a normal amount of anger and instead acts "holier than thou" and "thinks he's so perfect" even though he yells at the kids too sometimes. And on it goes.

Meanwhile I am listening to the words and the feelings, trying to see things through each one's eyes in turn and feel my way into each one's inner world. I gradually sense the loneliness and pain under all the anger and vitriol: the pain of having the person you love, depend on, and need to be loved by, criticising you, hating you, and not understanding you. I also note each one's complete lack of empathy for the other's position, and the attack-defend pattern, and the generous use they are making of the energising effects of righteous indignation – all the while wondering where, when, and how I might interrupt in a way that would feel empathic to both without it feeling to Will that I am just like all those previous therapists.

Finally, I hear myself saying in a dry, slightly humorous tone, that at the risk of sounding like one of those "family systems therapists," which I'm not really or solely (Will looks startled but bemused at this, and I see that he's ok with my use of humour here), and that while I'm not saying they are equally responsible for any particular behaviour or interaction, I do feel pretty equally badly for both of them. (I glance at Will here to see how that is going over. He seems wary but ok.) I tell them I understand how absolutely essential it feels for Will that Andrea expresses anger differently, gives him feedback in a more contained, less emotional way, and takes responsibility without excuses when she doesn't. And how essential it feels to Andrea that Will understands her behaviour in context without shaming her for it, and that she feel loved and understood and supported and not spoken to in a superior or condescending way. I say that the intensity with which they are each arguing their respective positions – and how long and hard they've been trying to get the other to change – tells me how important the other and their relationship must be to them, or at least must have been at one time. I say I think they are both emotionally malnourished in their marriage, but that, to their credit, they are both fighting hard for more emotional nutrition. They're nodding, and seeing that they are with me, I add that unfortunately the ways they are currently going about this are back-firing, but that there are other options that might work better.

This formulation seems to give both food for thought (an emotional nutrient) and to fit well enough that the mood in the room quietens. Both agree that the word malnourished is a good description and say they do feel they are fighting for their rights in a way, or for their emotional survival. Eventually, on a hunch, I say that while I think no spouse would appreciate explosive outbursts from their partner, and that anyone would want the one having them to admit responsibility and not make excuses, I'm also wondering if this might be an especially important need of Will's – maybe something he especially needs in order to be able to admire and respect his partner and feel close and safe. I can see in his eyes that I am right, or at least getting warm, so I gently ask if Andrea is the first person in his life who didn't meet that need. Again I see that I'm on the right track, but that this line of questioning is of course feeling dangerous to him. So I quickly say something like, "Uh oh, I just sounded like one of those typical shrinks there, didn't I, asking about your childhood when we haven't even addressed Andrea's behaviour yet? Are you feeling, like, oh, geez, here we go again?"

I can see this is a bullseye before he even confirms verbally, "You're damn right, that's exactly what I was thinking, and I'm telling you,

I'm not going through that again." I hold his gaze, receiving his anger and conveying my regret and apologies silently, through our eye dialogue, when after a minute he surprises us all, I think, by saying that actually I am right, he does need Andrea to be accountable and self-reflective partly because his parents were so abusive and out of control and never took responsibility for or apologised for anything. I will later learn that both parents are severe alcoholics who were routinely physically abusive to each other and their children during Will's upbringing, and continue to be extremely self-focused, massively misattuned, and often significantly verbally abusive to him to this day, despite now living across the country from the couple.

After a minute, I quietly ask Andrea how it feels to hear that part of the reason Will fights so hard to get her to admit wrong-doing and reacts so intensely when he feels she's minimising is because it feels so familiar, so close to old pain. To my relief, she softens and agrees that her in-laws are very limited, difficult people who never apologise or take responsibility for anything they do, and says she never wants to be anything like them or remind Will of them. Seeing that she's in a much more empathic place, I suggest that she turn to Will and say that again, right to him. She hesitates but does so, which Will clearly appreciates, and he responds by clarifying that he's not saying she's that much like them, which she appreciates. We discuss this further and eventually I point out how different, more nourishing, and gentler this dialogue feels compared to the one they were having earlier in the session. I say it looks like helping them have more of these kinds of empathic, gentler, more connected conversations, and fewer of the other kind, would be a major goal of our work, and they nod their agreement.

At this point we are nearing the end of the session and I notice I'm picturing the two of them reverting to their usual ways of relating by the time they get to their car. Following another hunch, I ask how much they know about the science of anger. Both look puzzled and convey some interest and curiosity, so I go into a little spiel about the body's fight or flight reflex in response to the perception of threat, whether physical or psychological. I explain its effects on the body (for example, release of adrenaline, increased heart rate, respiration rate, muscle tension, etc.), including the reduced activation of the brain's prefrontal cortex, the part of our brains that handles executive functions like logical, rational thinking, seeing things from multiple perspectives, and problem-solving. I say that's why people say things like, "I lost my mind" about times when they felt really angry or threatened, because actually they did, in a way.

Both seem intrigued. Andrea says, "Oh, so *that's* what's happening to me!" We talk for a few minutes about how this fits for her, and I eventually add that scientists have found that once adrenaline has been released, it can take 25–30 minutes for it to dissipate (Gottman, 1999) and for the prefrontal cortex to "come back online." I say this means we now have scientific support for the commonsense suggestion to take a time out when angry. A cardinal rule of good conflict resolution, therefore, is not to try to do it while either party is under the influence of a fight or flight reaction, because you need your prefrontal cortex to have any hope of a reasonable empathic dialogue – the kind of dialogue Will is asking for when he says he can take critical feedback if it's said nicely. I see that Will is still wary, concerned that this amounts to another type of excuse, but he likes the time out idea, seems comforted that I am giving them something educational or concrete, and readily makes another joint appointment.

This is the beginning of a complicated treatment that will involve weekly and sometimes twice weekly sessions for the next three years, continue intermittently for years after that, and cover many aspects of their relationship, starting with Andrea's angry outbursts but later expanding to conflicts about parenting, sex, money, and division of labour, all while they process or re-process their respective painful histories. Regardless of topic, the focus will be on helping them listen carefully and differently, understand in more complex and nuanced ways why they feel and act as they do, repair ruptures between them much more quickly and effectively, and have more fun together. Overall, they will come to function as a more reliable source of selfobject experience for each other.

Andrea will make great use of the idea of paying close attention to her level of physiological arousal before trying to confront anyone or have a conversation, which is a completely new idea for her despite her previous career in a health-related field. Along with other ideas and insights, it will help her immediately reduce and eventually completely stop her dysregulated outbursts, to Will's enormous relief. She will also come to understand and reduce her compulsivity, workaholism, and perfectionism, which will drop considerably once she feels securely attached to both me and Will, and once these behaviours have been repeatedly understood as ill-fated attempts to elicit needed selfobject responsiveness and meet her valid needs for self-esteem and connection. They will also decrease significantly once we work on making sure she gets adequate sleep, exercise, and down time, which I learned early on that she hasn't had in years.

After insisting for the first several months of the treatment that he'd already successfully processed his trauma history in a previous individual therapy, which he had found very powerful and helpful, Will gradually recognised that despite this excellent work, there was still more left to do around the ways his relationship with Andrea triggered or reactivated this history. He came to see that this additional work could not have been done in that individual treatment, as it required the additional information only available in the couple treatment modality (Leone, 2013b). During our work, with Andrea's support, Will became increasingly able to confront his parents on their continuing alcoholism and hurtful behaviour, and he eventually successfully distanced from them when it became clear that was best. His pedantic, superior attitude largely faded.

Over the course of the therapy, both partners came to see themselves and each other as people with good self-esteem in many areas, but what we came to call "pockets" of shaky or low self-esteem in others – pockets that could be pierced or tapped into by the other (and others) at times, leading to intense emotional reactions. We surfaced and examined other core organising principles, such as Will's belief that "healthy, mature adults express anger only in very calm, contained ways," and illuminated and gradually altered their cycles of mutual misattunements and selfobject failures. Some of these changes occurred due to insights developed through the collaborative process of understanding and explaining, some through explicit psycho-education and coaching by me, and most through the corrective aspects of their individual relationships with me, and eventually with each other.

## Discussion

This description of an initial session and the subsequent therapy illustrates many aspects of a Self Psychological approach to couple therapy, as well as the selective integration of psycho-education into a fundamentally psychoanalytic treatment. It illustrates, first, my efforts to immerse myself equally in each partner's subjective experience and respond with balanced empathic attunement to each, even when this required intentionally re-righting myself when one partner's experience was initially much easier for me to grasp and resonate with. It also shows my efforts to gently translate the couple's presenting complaints into the language of unmet selfobject needs, such as Will's need to admire, respect and feel safe with his wife, and Andrea's need to feel loved, understood, and treated respectfully by him. It also illustrates the value of focusing first on the forward edge of problematic behaviours – such as viewing arguing and bickering as desperate efforts to feel heard and understood and to stand up for themselves and their emotional needs – as well as the value of tentative, experience-near interpretations of the possible "trailing edge" origins of behaviour. Perhaps most important, the session demonstrates the crucial importance of vigilantly monitoring each partner's moment-to-moment experience of the session, including their sense of self and sense of connection. It shows the value of "sniffing out" and quickly addressing potential injuries or empathic ruptures, such as when I guessed that Will might be feeling that I was making excuses for Andrea or behaving too much like previous disappointing therapists. Were it not for that, the ensuing treatment might not have happened, as Will might not have returned.

Finally, the case example illustrates how the judicious use of psycho-education can be experienced as an attuned selfobject response that facilitates deeper connection between the partners. The "science of anger" information introduced a different understanding of Andrea's angry outbursts for both partners. It gently perturbed Will's entrenched view of Andrea's outbursts as immature, self-indulgent, or the result of Andrea not trying hard enough, and Andrea's only partially conscious belief that she was entitled to or justified in the occasional dysregulated outburst if sufficiently provoked. It also began to establish me as a knowledgeable expert with something to offer them – a potentially idealisable other who could be leaned on for strength and guidance, something that it turned out neither had had in their families. It is important to note that I introduced the psycho-education only when I sensed the couple might benefit from and appreciate the information, and continued with it only after watching closely and seeing that both seemed to find the information interesting and useful – or were experiencing it as an attuned selfobject response.

# Conclusion

Self Psychology offers a wealth of concepts that can be very useful to therapists struggling with the many challenges of couple therapy. Using Kohut's concept of selfobject experience as the image of what we are trying to promote, both between the partners and between ourselves and each partner, couple therapists can investigate and address the multiple factors that are interfering with couples' abilities to relate that way. Self Psychology's emphasis on the centrality of the patient's sense of self, sense of connection, and conscious affective experience; its view of the forward and trailing edges of behaviour; and its treatment approach involving sustained empathic immersion, balanced attuned responsiveness, collaborative, experience-near exploration and interpretation, close attention to narcissistic vulnerability and the rupture and repair sequence, and a recognition that selfobject relationships can be healing or change-promoting in themselves, all have important implications for couples treatment.

# References

Bacal, H. (1985). Optimal responsiveness and the therapeutic process. In A. Goldberg (Ed.), *Progress in self psychology*, Vol. 1, pp. 202–227. Hillsdale, NJ: Analytic Press.

Bacal, H. (Ed.). (1998). *Optimal responsiveness: How therapists heal their patients.* New York: Jason Aronson, Inc.

Boston Change Process Study Group (2008). Forms of relational meaning: Issues in the relations between the implicit and reflective/verbal dimensions. *Psychoanaltyic Dialogues, 18*, 125–148.

Fonagy, P., & Target, M. (1997). Attachment and reflective function: Their role in self organization. *Development and Psychopathology, 9*(4), 679–700.

Fonagy, P., Gergely, G., Jurist, E., & Target, M. (2004). *Affect regulation, mentalization, and the development of the self.* New York: Other Press.

Fosshage, J. L. (2005) The explicit and implicit domains in psychoanalytic change. *Psychoanalytic Inquiry, 25*, 516–539.

Geist, R. A. (2008). Connectedness, permeable boundaries, and the development of the self: Therapeutic implications. *International Journal of Psychoanalytic Self Psychology, 3*, 129–152.

Geist, R. A. (2009). Empathy, connectedness, and the evolution of boundaries in self psychological treatment. *International Journal of Psychoanalytic Self Psychology, 4*, 165–180.

Geist, R. A. (2010). Empathizing with Oedipus: A connectedness perspective. *International Journal of Psychoanalytic Self Psychology, 5*(4), 467–482.

Geist, R. A. (2011). The forward edge, connectedness, and the therapeutic process. *International Journal of Psychoanalytic Self Psychology, 6*(2), 235–251.

Geist, R. A. (2013). How the empathic process heals: A microprocess perspective. *International Journal of Psychoanalytic Self Psychology, 8*(3), 265–281.

Geist, R. A. (2016). From self-protection to relational protectiveness: The modification of defensive structures. *International Journal of Psychoanalytic Self Psychology*, *8*(3), 265–281.

Geist, R. A. (2020). Interpretation as carrier of selfobject functions: Catalyzing inborn potential. *Psychoanalysis, Self and Context*, *15*(4), 338–347. DOI: 10.1080/24720038.2020.1791127

Gottman, G. (1999). *The marriage clinic: A scientifically-based marital therapy*. New York: W.W. Norton.

Herzog, B. (2011). Procedural interpretation: A method of working between the lines in the nonverbal realm. *Psychoanalytic Inquiry*, *31*(5), 462–474. DOI: 10.1080/07351690.2011.552050

Kohut, H. (1959). Introspection, empathy, and psychoanalysis. *Journal of the American Psychoanalytic Association*, *7*, 459–483.

Kohut, H. (1971). *The analysis of the self: A systematic approach to the psychoanalytic treatment of narcissistic personality disorders*. New York: International Universities Press.

Kohut, H. (1977). *The restoration of the self*. New York: International Universities Press.

Kohut, H. ([1981] 2010). On empathy. *International Journal of Psychoanalytic Self Psychology*, *5*(2), 122–131. DOI: 10.1080/15551021003610026

Kohut, H. (1984). *How does analysis cure?* Chicago, IL: University of Chicago Press.

Lachmann, F. (2016). Credo. *Psychoanalytic Dialogues*, *26*(5), 499–512. DOI: 10.1080/10481885.2016.1214460

Leone, C. (2008). Couple therapy from the perspective of Self Psychology and intersubjectivity theory. *Psychoanalytic Psychology*, *25*(1), 79–98.

Leone, C. (2013a). Helping couples heal from infidelity: A self psychological, intersubjective perspective. *International Journal of Psychoanalytic Self Psychology*, *8*(3), 282–308.

Leone, C. (2013b). The unseen spouse in individual therapy: Pitfalls and possibilities for the individual therapist. *Psychoanalytic Dialogues*, *23*(3), 324–339.

Leone, C., & MacIntosh, H. (2013). Forms and transformations of connectedness in couples: How Self Psychology and "Emotionally Focused Therapy" can inform each other. Panel presented at the 36th Annual International Conference on the Psychology of the Self, Chicago, IL.

Leone, C. (2018). Response to MacIntosh's review and discussion of the psychoanalytic couple therapy journal literature: A self psychological, intersubjective perspective. *Psychoanalytic Inquiry*, *38*(5), 387–398. DOI: 10.1080/07351690.2018.1469904

Leone, C. (2019). When couple therapy has started but an affair is continuing: Key clinical moments, curative factors and lucky breaks in a self psychological couples treatment and its context. *Psychoanalysis, Self and Context*, *15*(2), 152–169. DOI: 10.1080/24720038.2019.1647209

Livingston, M. (1995). A self psychologist in couplesland: A multisubjective approach to transference and countertransference-like phenomena in marital relationships. *Family Process*, *34*(4), 427–439.

Livingston, M. (1998). Conflict & aggression in couples therapy: A self psychological vantage point. *Family Process*, *37*(3), 311–321.

Livingston, M. (2001a). Couples in the playspace: Self Psychology, dreams and couple therapy. *Journal of Couples Therapy*, *10*(3/4), 111–129.

Livingston, M. (2001b). *Vulnerable moments: Deepening the therapeutic process in individual, couples and group psychotherapy*. Northvale, NJ: Jason Aronson Press.

Livingston, M. (2007). Sustained empathic focus, intersubjectivity, and intimacy in the treatment of couples. *International Journal of Psychoanalytic Self Psychology*, *2*(3), 315–338.

Lyons-Ruth, K., Stern, D., Sander, L., Nahum, J., Harrison, A., Morgan, A., Bruschweiler-Stern, N., & Tronick, E. Z. (1998). Implicit relational knowing: Its role in development and psychoanalytic treatment. *Infant Mental Health Journal*, *19*, 282–289.

Lyons-Ruth, K. (1999). The two-person unconscious: Intersubjective dialogue, enactive relational representation, and the emergence of new forms of relational organization. *Psychoanalytic Inquiry*, *19*(4), 576–617.

MacIntosh, H. (2019). *Developmental couple therapy for complex trauma: A manual for therapists*. New York and London: Routledge.

Miller, J. (1985). How Kohut actually worked. In A. Goldberg (Ed.), *Progress in self psychology*, Vol. 1, pp. 13–30. New York: Guilford Press.

Mitchell, S. A., & Aron, L. (Eds.). (1999). *Relational perspectives book series, Vol. 14. Relational psychoanalysis: The emergence of a tradition*. Hillsdale, NJ: Analytic Press.

Pizer, B., & Pizer, S. (2006). The gift of an apple or the twist of an arm. *Psychoanalytic Dialogues*, *16*, 71–92.

Ringstrom, P. A. (1994). An intersubjective approach to conjoint therapy. In Arnold Goldberg (Ed.), *A decade of progress: Progress in self psychology*, Vol. 10, pp. 159–182. Hillsdale, NJ: Analytic Press.

Ringstrom, P. A. (2012). A relational psychoanalytic approach to conjoint treatment. *International Journal of Psychoanalytic Self Psychology*, *7*(1), 85–111.

Ringstrom, P. A. (2014). *A relational psychoanalytic approach to couples psychotherapy*. New York and London: Routledge.

Ringstrom, P. A. (2018). A relational psychoanalytic perspective of couples psychotherapy. *Psychoanalytic Inquiry*, *38*(5), 399–408.

Sander, L. (1991). Recognition process: Specificity and organization in early human development. Paper presented at University of Massachusetts conference, The Psychic Life of the Infant. As cited in Lyons-Ruth, K. (2000). I sense that you sense that I sense … Sander's recognition process and the specificity of relational moves in the psychotherapeutic setting. *Infant Mental Health Journal*, *21*(1–2), 85–98.

Sandmeyer, J. (2019). Understanding homophobia in our forefathers: Rethinking how Kohut actually worked. *Psychoanalysis, Self and Context*, *14*(4), 376–392.

Shaddock, D. (1998). *From impasse to intimacy: How understanding unconscious needs can transform relationships*. Northvale, NJ: Jason Aronson Press.

Shaddock, D. (2000). *Contexts and connections: An intersubjective approach to couples therapy*. New York: Basic Books.

Solomon, M. (1988). Treatment of narcissistic vulnerabilities in marital therapy. In A. Goldberg (Ed.), *Learning from Kohut: Progress in self psychology*, Vol. 4, pp. 215–230. Hillsdale, NJ: Analytic Press.

Stern, S. (2017). *Needed relationships and psychoanalytic healing: A holistic relational approach*. Abingdon-on-Thames: Routledge.

Stolorow, R., Brandshaft, B., & Atwood, G. (1987). *Psychoanalytic treatment: An intersubjective approach*. Hillsdale, NJ: Analytic Press.

Tolpin, M. (2002). Doing psychoanalysis of normal development: Forward edge transferences. In A. Goldberg (Ed.), *Progress in Self Psychology*, Vol. 18, pp. 167–190. Hillsdale, NJ: Analytic Press.

Trop, J. L. (1994). Conjoint therapy: An intersubjective approach. In A Goldberg (Ed.), *Progress in self psychology*, Vol. 10 (pp. 147–158). Hillsdale, NJ: Analytic Press.

Trop, J. (1997). An intersubjective perspective on countertransference in couple therapy. In M. Solomon, & J. Siegel (Eds.), *Countertransference in couple therapy* (pp. 99–109). Hillsdale, NJ: Analytic Press.

Weiss, M. (2018). Ethical presence in the psychoanalytic encounter and the role of apology. *The American Journal of Psychoanalysis*, 78(1), 28–46.

Winnicott, D. W. (1953). Transitional objects and transitional phenomena—A study of the first not-me possession. *International Journal of Psycho-Analysis*, 34(2), 88–97.

# Chapter 16

# Discussion of "The application of contemporary Self Psychology to couple psychotherapy"

*Rachel Cooke*

In her chapter, "The application of contemporary Self Psychology to couple psychotherapy," Carla Leone lays out a clear and comprehensive introduction to how she works with couples. She draws mainly on Self-Psychological theory, though she acknowledges having at her disposal a particular integration of various psychoanalytic and non-psychoanalytic ideas and techniques. In my discussion, I will look more closely at some of the ways in which the ideas she uses both converge with a contemporary object relations perspective, and where these ideas diverge.

Leone's paper presents an interesting opportunity to compare and differentiate what those of us formed in the crucible of the Tavistock model do, in contrast to her primarily Self-Psychological orientation, which derives mostly from Kohut and contemporary Self Psychology. Tavistock theory, by contrast, is not an integrative model, but hues closely to the evolution of British Object Relations theory. Until recently, at least, it has drawn exclusively from that history, primarily from Freud, Klein, Bion, the contemporary Kleinians (Ron Britton and John Steiner), and from the Tavistock clinicians at their couple relationship study unit, most importantly, Mary Morgan and James Fisher. The Tavistock model offers ways of applying traditional and contemporary psychoanalytic theory to working with couples. This means taking up theories of the unconscious and unconscious phantasy, transference and repetition, projection, and projective identification, the paranoid-schizoid and depressive positions, and crucially, narcissism. In the Tavistock model, these theories are specifically developed for use with couples, rather than with individuals.

In order to draw attention to some of the differences between the two approaches, I would like to offer a brief note on the history of

DOI: 10.4324/9781003265023-16

Self Psychology within the context of its evolution out of classical psychoanalytic theory. Self Psychology grew out of the work of Heinz Kohut, who made his home in Chicago, where his ideas took the firmest root (so it is no coincidence that Leone lives and works there). Like Freud and Melanie Klein before him, Kohut was a secular, upper-middle-class, assimilated Jew from Vienna, who emigrated under the inauspicious conditions of the Holocaust. Kohut was interested in a problem which presented in certain of his analytic patients, those with a comparatively narcissistic psychological structure. For Kohut, the problem was that these patients could not develop a transference to the analyst in the usual way, and this hampered the progress of the analytic work. For Freud, the transference was the heart of any treatment, and he also noticed that some patients, especially narcissistic patients, did not form a dependent attachment or transference to the analyst. Kohut's response to this problem was to develop a theory and practice which attempted to address directly how the analyst and his narcissistic patient might overcome such a barrier to the progress of the treatment. In classical Freudian theory, the only way the analyst might hope to cure the narcissist was to "somehow pry the self-directed libido out of its defensive, narcissistic orientation, and back into a more mature, outwardly directed channel" (Mitchell and Black, 1996, p. 153). Kohut rejected the notion that "prying" interpretation alone could bring about change. He thought interpretation led patients, especially the narcissistically vulnerable ones, to feel criticised or judged, and to become silently worse or dismissively angry. This in turn led to patients providing compliant solutions or quitting treatment altogether. Kohut sensed that there had to be a better way to help the narcissistic patient move beyond the limits of their otherwise walled off stance, their tendency towards grandiosity, and their thin-skinned self-absorption. Kohut viewed narcissism as a stalled developmental process, and he thought that the missing component by which to spur development was the analyst's empathic attunement (Kohut, 1959, 1979). The analyst's attunement was to be expressed, in part, by a willingness to wait for the transference to unfold, and by deferring the urge to make interpretations.

Kohut also contributed a new way of thinking about the transference. In place of the classical transference, he conceived of the "selfobject" transference, and he theorised that this was the key element of therapeutic change. Leone describes how the selfobject transference is established by the therapist's attempts to meet the patient's selfobject needs. Selfobject needs are those ordinary relational needs for recognition, understanding, and support. The development of a felt connection between patient and analyst brings about mirroring, idealising, and twinship transferences. Where Freud and Klein had offered interpretations (which could have an alienating effect), Kohut offered empathic recognition of the patient's wishes and capacities and encouragement for the patient to feel "mirrored," In this way, the patient would be more likely to feel equal to the analyst, rather than inferior or in competition with him. Only by assiduously meeting the selfobject needs of the patient, and by providing a meticulous brand of "empathic immersion" (Kohut, 1959), would the narcissist evolve. If Kohut's most important contribution to psychoanalytic technique was to make the analyst's empathy foundational in any treatment, then his theory of selfobject transference was the vehicle by which patients were understood and encouraged to seek it.

In her clinical application of Kohut's ideas to working with couples, Leone describes the selfobject needs and failures that inevitably occur between partners in couple relationships. As she discussed, the term "selfobject" describes any experience that feels affirming, "one that increases the felt sense of being understood" (Leone, this volume, p. 191). Of course, there are inevitable ruptures in the connection and goodwill which lead couples to therapy, but Leone's aim is to help the couple develop this ability, no matter the intensity of the ruptures they present with. For Leone, one main goal of the couple therapist is to help each member of the couple expand their capacity to meet their partner's selfobject needs. As part of this process, she models the capacity to attend to each person's attunement needs with careful consistency. In each session, she is also hoping to score a "bullseye," a comment that feels exactly right to her patients, one which constitutes a gratifying moment of connection for patient and couple therapist alike (Leone, this volume, p. 195).

Leone also elaborates the bedrock quality of her empathic attunement. As a Self Psychologist, she provides a stance of "equal empathic immersion into each partner's subjective affective experience" (Leone, this volume, p. 195). Empathic connection has a particular importance in couple work because, in some ways, it's much more exposing and frightening to come in for treatment with a partner than on one's own.

Much of the sense of danger that couples often feel when starting couple therapy stems from the fact that neither partner knows what the other is going to say, or what they might express to the therapist. Listening to Leone's approach, we can hear how hard she works to be attuned and responsive to her couples, and to help them feel safe. I think this stance is behind her saying, "in every session, my goal first and foremost is for each partner to feel deeply understood and empathically responded to by me – before I worry about trying to help them understand things differently" (Leone, this volume, p. 195). She demonstrates this approach in the case example of Will and Andrea, by attempting to make a good selfobject connection with each of them separately at the outset. I agree with Leone and think this sort of care is an essential provision for any couple treatment to proceed.

Being a part of a couple is not easy and it requires being psychological to navigate the anxieties and stresses that can arise. Leone's "bullet" list of psychological capacities (Leone, this volume, p. 192–193) is very thorough, offering a comprehensive set of qualities that describe a state of psychological maturity. She refers specifically to the importance of having "a positive, cohesive sense of self," as opposed to "a shaky, or negative sense of self" (ibid, p. 192–193). She writes that Kohut believed that a "positive... sense of self was central to psychological health and adaptive functioning" (ibid, p. 192–193). Although this belief is a useful starting point, I think it leaves a lot of territory uncharted, and stops short of a necessary and much more detailed theorisation of the psychological substrate of the individual and the couple. In my view, the Tavistock model offers a deeper understanding of the level of psychological functioning of each member of the couple, as well as of the couple together. Leone also seems to recognise the limits of what Self Psychology has to offer. Her use of affect regulation theory, and of Fonagy and Target's work on mentalisation (ibid, p. 193) show how she thinks beyond Self Psychology. Indeed, she openly acknowledges her approach is eclectic.

## British Object Relations theory and the Tavistock model of working with couples

Hailing as it does from a long line of British Object Relations theorists, the Tavistock model consists of a many-tiered psychoanalytic approach to working with couples. This kind of psychoanalytic approach takes the key components of object relations theory and applies them to working with couples. It privileges the unconscious dimension. It offers a way of noticing and speaking to the projective systems at work in the couple and to the inevitability of unconscious patterns of repetition. It helps therapists learn to listen for the shared unconscious layers that inhabit the couple and bring these to light by offering intricate observations about the ways in which couples' beliefs coexist and overlap. It uses the ideas of the depressive and paranoid-schizoid positions to distinguish between levels of psychological functioning.

Leone's description of the well-developed capacities couples need to achieve in order to meet each other's selfobject needs roughly correlates with the idea of the depressive position, yet there isn't a theorisation of the more disturbed side of the personality. When the paranoid-schizoid position predominates, it gives rise to all sorts of misguided or hateful beliefs about the self and the other. In the paranoid-schizoid position, people are liable to be reactive, to shut down and go on the attack. In this state, partners cling to partial truths as certainties, blame each other, and claim to be in possession of "the" truth. At its most intense, working with couples requires spending a lot of time grappling with the false certainties each person carries around about the other, and trying to loosen their grip.

## Narcissistic relating

In these extremely fraught situations, projections are rife between partners and the degree of narcissistic relating intensifies. Narcissistic object relating has been well theorised in the Tavistock model (Ruszczynski and Fisher, 1995; Fisher, 1999). Although narcissism exists on a continuum and can be mild or severe, one of its central features is the denial of the other person's separate and independent being. An individual might make assumptions about their partner in an ordinary narcissistic moment, but at the other end of the spectrum they might be relentless in their refusal to allow or accept the other person's experience. These refusals are characterised by attempts to control the other person either directly or by means of evacuative projections. Narcissistic object relating describes a state of psychic blindness consisting of a lack of curiosity and a refusal of the other's independent emotional existence, or an overall intolerance of the other as *other* at all. Because it consists of (mostly unconscious) efforts to exert control over the other person, it leads to the belief that one knows what is in the other's mind without having to ask. There is a high degree of overlap between narcissistic states and the para-noid-schizoid position, meaning that both are primitive states of mind in which partners are likely to be blaming and accusing or demanding of perfect attunement.

James Fisher (1999), a central contributor to the Tavistock litera-ture on couples, proposed that narcissism is precisely opposite to a "psychological state of marriage." At best, there are lifelong oscilla-tions between states of narcissistic relating on one hand and object relating on the other, just as there are continual shifts back and forth between the depressive and paranoid-schizoid positions in couple relating. Fisher writes that narcissism is "a longing for an other who is perfectly attuned and responsive, and thus not a genuine other at all" (Fisher, 1999, pp. 1–2). The wish for perfect attunement is an infantile wish which returns at moments across the lifespan but exists as more of a continuous demand in someone with a narcissistic structure. Thus, where as "the psychological state of 'marriage'" is informed by curiosity and the capacity to make room for two, the state of narcis-sism refuses to look outside of itself and insists that there is only room for one. I think this raises some important questions for technique in working with such couples. Does the self-psychological emphasis on empathic attunement give the narcissist a little too much of what they already believe they are entitled to? Is it possible that by accommodat-ing the narcissist to such a degree, the therapist only exacerbates these tendencies? Or is it the case that sensitive attunement to these needs is the only way to help develop the capacity to accept the full existence of someone else? When working with couples who are more narcissis-tically or primitively organised, I think it is possible to make progress by means of a careful balance of both empathic attunement and gen-tle, kind confrontation of some of these demands.

Here's an example of working with narcissistic self-absorption in this way. A heterosexual couple, both in their second marriage and neither with children, were in a fight over whose parents they would spend the upcoming holidays with. With one set of parents in the east coast and the other in Southern California, it would not be possible to visit both. The man insisted that they would visit his parents, as usual, for Christmas. The woman protested that they've visited his parents each year for the five years of their marriage, and that she would like to visit her parents for a change. Ordinarily they spent Thanksgiving with her parents but this year, for various reasons, that would not be possible. The man would not be moved. He declared that the custom is to stay with his family for Christmas, and that his parents want to see him very much. He said this with great emphasis. The woman took a deep breath and (seeming to pluck up her courage), suggested to her husband that her parents too, would like to see their daughter for Christmas. The man appeared uncomprehending and said that he wanted to see his parents. The therapist attempted to point out the man's assumption that they would both do what he wanted to do each year, with which he readily agreed. Then the therapist gently questioned this assumption. How come he expected this? "We have always done it this way," he said definitively, as if it were an agreed upon tradition that allowed for no revision and ignored the legitimacy of his wife's or her parents' desires.

Most of the time the couples who come for treatment are not extreme narcissists, and though many do fall on the narcissistic continuum, by far the most frequent and ordinary examples of narcissistic object relating occur in the context of unconscious projective systems. Couples often project the negatively installed parts of their own, or someone else's personality, in a way that tends to repeat aspects of early, formative relationships. Thus, there is considerable overlap between moments of narcissistic relating and their unconscious projections into each other. Fights commonly erupt in this way.

Here's a brief example of an ordinary projective interaction, a fight which starts in an apparently benign and ordinary moment and is common in non-narcissistically organised couples. The work involves helping each member of the couple realise that the disruptive dynamic between them is co-created and the product of deeply structured anxieties that interact projectively between them. Mario and Thomas are a young, married gay couple. Mario came home, tired from work. Thomas was making burgers for dinner. When Mario looked in the pan, he saw that Thomas had shaped the burgers into squares rather than circles, and in his tired and hungry state, Mario irritably questioned the choice of making the meat into a square shape when the buns they were using were round. Thomas looked up and angrily snapped, "What's wrong with that?" He escalated the situation, demanded that Mario tell him about the problem with his decision, stormed out of the kitchen and threatened to not finish preparing dinner. Mario took a deep breath, apologised, and told Thomas not to worry about it.

Their bad feelings resolved after they ate dinner, but the incident had unsettled Mario enough to bring the episode into couple therapy, to take a closer look at what might have happened below the surface. Mario insightfully said he had felt less upset about the shape of the burger than over Thomas' immediate reactive anger towards him. Mario realised he had wanted to be able to be irritated without Thomas getting reactive and angry. But instead, he felt that he had to be the one to back down and appease Thomas. He resented having to do that. This reminded me that Mario's moods were often questioned, or frankly disallowed, in his family of origin. He felt his mother had experienced him as a burden and had often required him to stifle his emotional responses. I pointed out how he lives with the belief that he is never allowed the emotional freedom to feel irritable or petulant, and that his husband had unwittingly confirmed this emotional truth by his intolerant reaction to his criticism of the burger.

On Thomas' side, I commented that he seemed to be excessively sensitive to Mario's comment about the shape of the burger. When I inquired who else in his life might have questioned his abilities or talked down to him, this poignantly led to a memory of his father. In the memory, his frequently absent father was visiting and playing ball with him. When Thomas hadn't been able to catch the ball, his father called him "useless" and refused to continue to play. At that moment, the link between this memory and his experience with Mario became clear. Since it felt to him that Mario was also calling him useless and stupid, it was no wonder he became defensive and enraged. After we spent some time reflecting on this, the couple were able to note how ridiculous it all was that neither of them had been able to have a playful or flexible response in such a superficially innocuous situation, and we were all able to laugh about it together.

This is what can happen between couples and wreaks havoc on an otherwise peaceable existence. Without either partner having conscious awareness of it, a fight is poised to erupt largely based on the unconscious, present-day misrecognition of each other as representing aspects of early relationship figures (usually parental figures). By shedding light on these separate but unconsciously overlapping origin stories, the therapist can help the couple understand what underlies their fight and reduce the likelihood of their continually falling into the same trap. It's important to uncover these projective patterns in order to help couples begin to be more psychologically separate, and to start to know themselves, and each other, more fully. This will help them avoid these types of projectively driven fights that can arise so instantly and can be so emotionally debilitating.

## Different technical considerations between the two models

In a previous version of her paper (given at the annual conference of PCPG/NCSPP, see Nathans and Schaefer, 2017, p. xiv), Leone included a footnote that offered a useful distinction between her orientation and my own. She suggested that the Self Psychologist implicitly asks, "What does the patient need from me?" Whereas the object-relational psychotherapist might be asking, "What's going on around here?" Leone is thinking primarily about how to meet her patients' needs, whereas I am actively trying to notice and describe what's happening *between* the members of the couple. I'm looking for and listening to the conscious, surface levels for what they say, but also attempting to get at what is not said, or what's so far out of consciousness that it's not speakable at all. I'm listening for elements of the transference repetition in order to help the couple build a map of how they unconsciously intersect. I'm noticing their affect and lack of it, their level of interest in each other, and the areas of similarity and difference between them. Leone is doing much of this too, although I think her emphasis falls elsewhere. She considers her presence as central to the couple, and her empathic attunement to each of them *separately* forms the body of her work until it is well established. As she states it, the focus is on the "corrective aspects of their individual relationships with *me*, and *eventually* with each other" (Leone, this volume, p. 205, italics mine).

In contrast, I go to work on the couple's relationship immediately. I go back and forth with each member of the couple, building alliances. Like Leone, I am always keeping an ear open for how each of the partners might be hearing me. For the most part, I address and think about them as a couple, aiming to make observations about their relationship, and attempting to hold a "couple state of mind" (Morgan, 2019). I might offer a kind of "paired" observation, one that seeks to delineate their experience at opposite poles of a spectrum. Once these emotional poles are stated, it can open up the possibility of determining the more reality-based middle ground. For instance, with one warring couple in my office this week, I said to the husband, "*You feel* accused of never doing enough"; and to the wife I said, "*You feel* he doesn't keep you in mind." The truth is usually somewhere in between. Each person contributes unconsciously to the tendency to believe the more extreme version is true. I also make "joint" interpretations addressed to the couple together, observations about the commonality of their experience, such as, "I think you both feel unsafe," or "There are two hurt people in the room," or "I think you both want to feel an intimate connection with each other, but you go about it in ways that the other person isn't receptive to." These kinds of statements serve as the gateway to in-depth conversations about aspects of their families of origin, other important relationships, and whatever else we can find in their emotional "infrastructure." This process leads towards a greater capacity for each to notice or acknowledge the experience of the other and to know the other more fully, as each wish to be known. This process isn't the same as Leone's, yet it's quite proximate to helping the couple better meet each other's selfobject needs.

Leone is clear that she positions herself as an expert where the couple are concerned. She does this in part to encourage their "idealising" needs, to support their belief that they are in good hands with her and will get the help they need. The Tavistock stance is different. I think we are more modest about our expertise, and less sure what the couple needs from us. Our expertise is implicit; bound up with the fact of their seeking out our professional help and guidance. We pursue with curiosity whatever the couple brings, and we try to sit in uncertainty until there's an observation to be made or a hunch about a pattern of some kind. We may think about how the couple are using us and what their conscious or unconscious ideas are about who we are to them (including negative or devaluing transferences), but we don't seek out the experience of creating an idealising transference as such. The history of our theory leaves us uncomfortable with idealisation since it's long been considered a defence. Devaluation is its flip side, and in paranoid-schizoid states, it can swing there very quickly.

Leone also shows a confidence in her way of talking with her couple that I think derives from her sense that she knows precisely what to offer, leading with empathy and cultivating selfobject transferences. I think confidence in the Tavistock model derives more from our ideas about containment and the containing function we offer our couples. This is our ability to make what Morgan calls, a "couple analytic space" (Morgan, 2019, p. 19), a place to which they are invited to bring any aspects of their relationship while we maintain at all times, to the best of our ability, a thoughtful, non-judgemental, balanced state of mind.

Similarly, in the Tavistock model, I don't think we view ourselves as central in the same way Leone does. Rather, we think of our role as a kind of "Uninvited Guest," (to quote Fisher quoting T.S. Eliot, Fisher, 1999), or at very least, the ambivalently invited guest of the anxious or stressed-out couple. One of our theoretical tenets is an interest in the psychological significance of inclusion and exclusion. Following Ron Britton (1989), who has theorised at length about the Oedipal Situation and triangular dynamics, we acknowledge our position as external to and excluded from the couple, and we aim to model a comfort with this. I believe it is because I'm comfortable being outside of the couple, and different from them, that I can have a couple state of mind, a position from which I can observe them. Without it, I could be seduced into forming an alliance with one member of the couple against the other. With it, I can step back and think about them separately and together, thereby modelling a vital reflective capacity. Morgan points out that this reflective capacity is sometimes missing in a couple, in which case they cannot "think about themselves as a couple" (Morgan, 2019, p. xxii). It's not just when emotions are flooding them that some couples can't think. They may be too entrenched in their deeply held misconceived beliefs about each other to step back and think about what they believe. In this way of working, we attempt to offer them our capacity to step back and think.

Leone also highlights the idea of the forward and trailing edge, which she writes is the second major contribution of Self Psychology to couple therapy. She elaborates how this often consists of someone trying to get a need met but going about it in a problematic way. This is also theorised in the Tavistock model, although the language is different. We say the couple is relating in defensive *and* developmental ways, and we try to track both. What may look like a developmental striving can also have regressive aims. Alternatively, an apparently defensive repetition can be an attempt to outgrow an old pattern.

Let's say my patient (in a young married couple), gets upset with his wife in the airplane coming home from a trip, because she wants to use the plane's WiFi, and he knows it's an "unsecured" network that will likely result in the theft of her personal information. His wife, also my patient, is upset, because she had the idea that they could be cosy and watch something together on her device. He insists she would be irresponsible to sign onto the network. As a result, she sulks. She deliberately turns away from him and falls asleep. He spends the flight feeling angry that he's the only responsible one in the couple, while she feels slighted, and controlled. He is controlling, yes, but is it all negative? I think Leone might notice his desire to protect her from some unidentified airborne hacker as a forward edge. Similarly, is her sulkiness regressive? Yes, but it also reasserts her separateness and refusal to accept being controlled without putting up a protest. It's not mature, and of course that needs to be addressed in the therapy, as does his controlling insistence that she keep her device switched off.

In the hour, I said to them, "You both wanted to be of one mind, you wanted to see the situation the same way, instead of two people, two minds." And the man, psychologically sophisticated in some ways, asked, "Why is it so hard to agree to disagree?" This is a man whose parents were very undependable. There was nothing "secure" there for him (remember the "unsecured" network). He got where he is in life by being rigorously effective and rational, so he can't tolerate the slightest hint of irrationality in his wife. She had a father who made no attempt to curb his meanness around her and who routinely cut her down to size, so that's a point of her particular vulnerability. All of us sitting in the room have come to know these layers over the few months of working together, so a moment like the fight on the plane provides insight into the bad kind of fit they're going to have to keep an eye on in order to prevent it from catching them unawares. As the mood lightened in the room, he said, "What about J-walking? Is that the same thing?" We realised that their levels of risk tolerance, so different, manifest even on the kerb of a city street as she pulls him into the street to cross and he says, "No, babe, let's go over to the crosswalk."

The couple therapist must work to help each member of the couple feel safe even as she asks them to give voice to what is most painful and adversarial in their relationship. So many people hold onto their hurts, unable to discuss them, and show up in couple therapy with years' worth of grudges and resentments. We try to get them talking, understanding they can't attempt these conversations at home, or if they try, things will rapidly go off the rails. Couples come to couple therapy to have the conversations they cannot have at home. Invariably these are stressful conversations, and it takes courage to have them. A conflict averse husband in a couple drew an analogy to scuba diving to illustrate his distaste for couple therapy. He explained that when scuba diving you have to glide along smoothly or else you stir up sand and silt, messing up the view of the underwater scene. He said, the trouble with these conversations is they keep kicking up sand. His wife responded that for her these conversations feel indispensable: talking in therapy helps filter out the silt and sand, offering hope for them to see each other clearly and connect lovingly again. A woman in another couple has referred to our sessions as being, "unpleasantly helpful." Comments like these illuminate the necessity for the therapist's deeply felt empathic register and attunement, but also the importance of helping the individual partners see beneath the surface, beyond what is consciously known.

In her case discussion, Leone is doing what she calls "collaborative empathic interpretation" with her couple patients. It's a great phrase, and I think it captures much of what I'm also doing in my work. Perhaps the differences are constituted by where the emphasis is in this aspect of the work. Namely, her emphasis on the centrality of the therapist and the therapist's empathic presence, the sense that she knows what her patients need from her, and the cultivation of their idealising transference, all are in the specific domain of Self Psychology. Thinking about projection, unconscious agreements, thirdness and difference are some of the object relations/Tavistock contributions. In both instances, there is attention to the transference repetition, a dedicated emphasis on listening to the couple, and doing whatever we can to improve their ability to listen to each other and accept points of view different from their own. This is the key: to transform the narcissistic refusals of unpleasant otherness into the willing acceptance of the other's experience, without either having to give up their own. I hope I have described some of the reasons why, contrary to our popular aphorism, it can be so very difficult to "live and let live."

# References

Britton, R. (1989) The missing link: Parental sexuality in the Oedipus Complex. In: J. Steiner (Ed.), *The Oedipus Complex today: Clinical implications* (pp. 83–101). London: Karnac.

Fisher, J. (1999) *The uninvited guest*. London: Karnac.

Kohut, H. (1959) Introspection, empathy and psychoanalysis. *Journal of the American Psychoanalytic Association*, 7(3): 459–483.

Kohut, H. (1979) The two analyses of Mr Z. *International Journal of Psychoanalysiss*, 60(3): 3–27.

Mitchell, S. and Black, M. (1996) *Freud and beyond: A history of modern psychoanalytic thought*. New York: Basic Books.

Morgan, M. (2019) *A couple state of mind*. London: Routledge.

Nathans, S. and Schaefer, M., eds. (2017) *Couples on the couch: Psychoanalytic couple therapy and the Tavistock Model*. London: Routledge.

Ruszczynski, S. and Fisher, J., eds. (1995) *Intrusiveness and intimacy in the couple*. London: Karnac.

# Chapter 17

# Co-parent therapy and the parenting plan as transitional phenomena[1]

## Working psychoanalytically with high-conflict separating and divorcing couples

*Dana Iscoff*

Significant challenges, including emotional turmoil and pervasive life changes, are at the heart of what is at stake in high-conflict separation and divorce. This paper focuses on the clinical and technical issues of working psychoanalytically with high-conflict separating and divorcing couples struggling with co-parenting issues. These parenting issues generally fall under the auspices of the family law system in the United States and are often managed through various psycho-educational interventions. My approach, which is based on psychoanalytic principles, extends a co-parenting/psycho-educational process to a deeper co-parent therapy, and takes the couple's level of psychological functioning into account. I offer a model, whereby the therapist helps the separating and divorcing couple develop a parenting plan while, at the same time, providing containment for the couple's anxieties about the separation or divorce. In my conception, the parenting plan may serve as a transitional object for the couple, facilitating their psychological development, and aiding in their transition from a separating or divorcing couple to a co-parent couple.

## Identifying high-conflict separating and divorcing couples

In separation and divorce, couples and their children may suffer profound disruptions in all aspects of their lives. They must manage changes in their identity, daily routines, and residences, as well as cope with the shifting bonds between parents, children, and networks of friends and family (Johnston & Campbell, 1988). Most importantly,

1 I would like to thank Dr Shelley Nathans for her support and her close reading of this paper.

DOI: 10.4324/9781003265023-17

couples going through separation and divorce must manage a complex array of intense feelings including loss, anger, guilt, betrayal, disappointment, and fear. Many couples are able to shield their children from the significant impact of these conflicts and disruptions, however, others cannot. When this occurs, it can result in interminable struggles and years of litigation with unrelenting conflicts over the children, negatively impacting them in both the short and the long term.

The psychodynamics of the couple, and the personality dynamics of the individuals, are the most prominent factors contributing to separation and divorce difficulties. Each partner brings their unconscious wishes, internal conflicts, and defences to the relationship to repair their internal and joint struggles (Nathans & Schaefer, 2017). The mutual fit of these projections, and the ability to recognise the other's separate reality, are essential for a healthy relationship. In contrast, high-conflict couples have difficulties in these domains, and a loss of hope in repairing early object relations exists. This unconscious dynamic pulls the partners into a relationship in which they have difficulty seeing one another as separate. Thus, they cannot cope with the subsequent feelings of anxiety, anger, and loss, and rely on primitive defences to evacuate and manage their pain.

Several authors have described the underlying dynamics of high-conflict couples from a psychoanalytic perspective. Bagnini (2003) characterised these relationships as attempts to repair early or lost objects, whereby the dissolution of the relationship can be experienced as another lost object, magnifying an already devastating loss from childhood. Lasso (2003) emphasised difficulties with separation anxiety and the defences against inevitable loss and mourning. This results in couples remaining united through conflict, causing the separation and divorce to remain incomplete and irresolvable. In this interminable divorce, partners continue to relate in a collusive manner, which in turn appears to prevent the pain of separation. Donner (2006) highlighted that some high-conflict separating and divorcing couples are extremely narcissistically vulnerable and overwhelmed by pathological amounts of envy. These couples are unable to think beyond their own emotional needs and must ward off their psychic collapse by fighting over custody even if it can result in harming and destroying their children.

Intense feelings of abandonment and the pain of early childhood traumatic separations can be activated in separating and divorcing couples. This can precipitate a repetition compulsion with a partner in an attempt to retaliate against a hurtful object and avoid mourning. Hatred dominates, the main goal is to destroy one another, and the motivation is to resist any resolution, sustaining the couple's conflicts (Demby, 2009).

## High-conflict separation and divorce in the US legal system

The legal system is often not equipped to deal with the conscious and unconscious behaviours of the co-parenting struggles of high-conflict couples and can be bewildering to judges and attorneys. Nevertheless, couples often seek help through the authority of the family law system to solve their impasses, and to contain and organise the circumstances of their entrenchment (Lasso, 2003). Judges and attorneys send many of these couples to mediation, where the goal is to make compromises and reach agreements. However, mediation assumes a certain psychological capacity. These couples, who are fighting about the care of their children, and embroiled in rigid defensive splitting, are less likely to access a state of mind in which they can reasonably make agreements – a necessary skill for mediation.

Alternatively, many separating and divorcing couples are sent by attorneys or the court to a clinician for co-parent counselling to help them create a parenting plan. The explicit goal is to have a legal document outlining the parenting schedules, policies, and responsibilities of shared parenting, based on the best interests of the children, and ostensibly towards the goal of reducing conflict and litigation. However, without considering the deeper unconscious conflicts of the couple, the parenting plan can be limited in its value to the couple and the children.

In other cases, the conflicts continue to escalate, sometimes for years, entangling parents and their children in turmoil, and requiring more contentious legal interventions. Judges may appoint a parenting coordinator to implement the policies of the parenting plan, to help reach agreements, and to make decisions when the parents are unable to do so. Additionally, the courts may order a child custody evaluation to assess the family's relationships and dynamics. In an evaluation, the child is seen as the prospective patient, and the goal is to understand how the parents support or interfere with the child's healthy physical and psychological development (Demby, 2009).

Paradoxically, the legal system, which can sometimes focus on who is the "better" parent in high-conflict separating and divorcing couples, often inadvertently promotes splitting and perpetuates the unconscious psychological collusion that caused the couples to become highly conflictual in the first place. Many family courts are limited in their capacity to deal with the unconscious motivations of the parents' perpetual conflicts that emerge among high-conflict couples. If the inability to mourn, and the pathological hatred of the other parent, become the primary motivating factors, then a circular pattern of conflict emerges, making the custody dispute the new relationship pattern (Levite & Cohen, 2011). This circular pattern causes the couple to remain psychologically stuck in a repetitive cycle of anger and blame, making the transition to becoming a co-parent couple difficult.

## Co-parent therapy

In my model of co-parent therapy, the therapist works with high-conflict couples to create a parenting plan, while at the same time, addressing the underlying psychological vulnerabilities contributing to their inability to separate and develop into a co-parent couple. While there is considerable overlap with other therapeutic approaches that use psychoanalytic concepts (e.g., Morgan, 2001; Nathans & Schaefer, 2017, Nyberg & Hertzmann, 2014), most of these approaches rely on the couple's motivation to come to therapy. High-conflict separating and divorcing couples are generally not motivated to participate in couple psychotherapy. In contrast, in my co-parent therapy model, the parenting plan serves as the motivating vehicle for the couples. Therefore, a different frame and technique is required. The work is aimed at delinking the couple as a relationship or marital couple, and at the same time, helping them form a new link as a co-parent couple. While the couple's impetus for coming to therapy is the development of the parenting plan, co-parent therapy addresses the psychodynamics that impede the development of the plan.

Psychologically, the couples in co-parent therapy are generally in a regressed state in which their external reality stimulates primitive internal reactions. They are often locked in bitter struggles, unable to stay together, but unable to separate emotionally, and persistently antagonise each other (Scharff, 2004). When such couples are so vehemently entrenched in their inability to tolerate their feelings and need to see one another as "bad," it is difficult to help the couple communicate and build a solid parenting agreement, even if it will protect the children from chaos, instability, and conflict.

High-conflict separating and divorcing couples often rely on defensive projective identification. They demonstrate, with varying degrees of severity, a profound inability to feel psychically separate from each other, and these differences are seen as persecutory. Morgan's (1995) concept of projective gridlock is helpful in understanding the complexity of these problematic dynamics. She described how couples, such as these, can be locked in a pathological projective identification, with the aim of denying another's separateness to the extent to which they each feel psychically captive. These couples cannot engage with one another, as *an other*, without feeling a threat to themselves. This defensive organisation allows the couple to attempt to get rid of intolerable feelings, experiences, and parts of the self, by projecting them into their partner. Evacuating these unwanted parts can then be defensively split off, relocated in the other, and identified with, from a distance.

Additionally, narcissistic vulnerability is one of the most common psychological manifestations in high-conflict couple relationships. Narcissism, and narcissistic vulnerabilities, are characterised by problems in the capacity to maintain a clear sense of identity, and the need for agreement is a primary aspect of the relating (Nathans & Schaefer, 2017; Ruszczynski, 1993). Battling over seemingly insignificant issues, devaluing the other parent, and fighting over child custody, are common in narcissistically organised high-conflict couples. Correspondingly, these couples have difficulty acknowledging or recognising their children's needs. They are motivated to primarily gratify their own needs, which ultimately is at the expense of the child (Donner, 2006). Furthermore, these types of couples cannot tolerate feelings of failure, humiliation, and shame. They often engage in varying degrees of distorted thinking and blame the other partner for the failure of the relationship. This results in severe despair and helplessness, whereby they vehemently strive for total control of their child and the ex-partner, in an attempt to ward off psychic collapse (Donner, 2006).

High-conflict couples often present with trouble differentiating in important domains of experience resulting in impediments to the development of the parenting plan and the co-parent therapy. First, their problems with psychic separation can result in an inability to distinguish between what is "me" and "not me" (Shmueli, 2005), and struggle to accept any differences between them. Secondly, they often have difficulty distinguishing between present and past experience and can become preoccupied and hold onto past resentments. Finally, there is often confusion between what belongs to their role as a couple and what belongs to their role as parents (Shmueli, 2005).

Since working with these high conflicts couples can be challenging, it can be useful for the therapist to maintain a "couple state of mind" (Morgan, 2001). This refers to the therapist's capacity to relate to each of the individual partners separately, while at the same time, relating to the couple relationship. This enables the therapist to work with projections, splitting, reality distortions, feelings of disappointment, anger, and grief over the lost relationship, and the transference and countertransference. In co-parent therapy, it is important for the therapist to recognise each of the partner's separate emotional experiences, and the impact on their relationship, while holding in mind the ways in which these experiences facilitate or interfere with the development of the plan.

Countertransference reactions are reflective of the intensity of each partner's struggles. The therapist may be experienced as an idealised, benevolent container, or as a judgemental, or persecutory, object. The couple's use of primitive defences can be challenging and demand that the therapist be drawn into the defensive system. It is difficult to avoid becoming enmeshed in the split and resist the immense pressure to be pulled into the experience of one individual at the expense of the other. Because projective identification is a common style of communication with these couples, enactments are often present. Working with these dysregulated couples will inevitably be manifested in the therapist's countertransference, but the greatest hazard is when this remains out of awareness (Nyberg & Hertzmann, 2019).

The therapist must provide a holding environment of a consistent and safe space without impingement; an active offering of insight and understanding for the difficult emotions and interactions (Ruszczynski, 1992). Interpreting unconscious internal processes may increase the couple's defensiveness because it can unrealistically force them to take back their own projections. Sometimes, it may be necessary for the therapist to focus on the more conscious aspects of the couple's experience (Shmueli, 2012). The therapist must help the couple track, identify, and recognise their irrational thinking, and the unresolved feelings of rage that resist developing insight (Donner, 2006). At other times, the therapist may be able to offer interpretations that address their deeper dynamics. This can be useful to help them to better understand their emotions, increase their capacity to think, and to be more reflective (Colman, 1993).

Offering guidance regarding the logistics of shared parenting is an important component of working on the development of the parenting plan. However, high-conflict couples can be so entrenched, escalating in their arguments, and unreflective that they are often unable to use the therapist's guidance. At times, direct, authoritative advice is required to shift their fused interlocking states in order to dislodge their defences and anxieties (Vincent, 2001). For example, in my work with a couple who argued about decisions regarding their 10-year-old child and could not agree on the merits of their child's psychotherapist, it was necessary to advise them against stopping the child's therapy. Recommending that they not make a rash decision was an important therapeutic intervention. However, therapists need to be aware that giving advice can also become an unconscious enactment within the therapy, which may interfere with the couple's process and look as if the therapist is aligning with one parent over the other (Vincent, 2001).

## The parenting plan

Despite the evidence that interpersonal cooperation is important for both the parents' and the children's well-being, very little has been written about the structure of the parenting plan, or the psychological dynamics associated with it (Ehrenberg & Hunter, 1996). The parenting plan is an individualised and detailed list of agreements, rules, and policies related to the parenting time schedule and shared parental responsibilities. In the best scenario, this can both guide and symbolise the newly formed co-parent couple. The successful ending of a relationship, or marriage, is often determined by what is created in its place (Clulow, 1990).The plan can mark the beginning of the couple's capacity to relate in a less persecutory and blaming way, and as it is internalised, it helps them transition to becoming a co-parent couple.

However, some couples will not be able to successfully use co-parent therapy or the parenting plan and will need to return to court for continued litigation. In other cases, they may not return to the courts and their conflicts will remain unchecked. It is sometimes necessary that parenting plans get developed by each individual's attorney or the family court. In these cases, the couple may not be actively involved in developing the plan. Instead, the plan is arrived at through legal negotiation. Therefore, the splitting and malignant projective processes may continue in the legal system. The history of unmitigated fighting, resentments, and extreme narcissistic vulnerability can prevent the psychological developmental work necessary to transition to a co-parent couple. Additionally, despite the legal intervention, the plan may be rejected, and its transitional possibilities rendered unusable.

For those who can use co-parent therapy, I am promoting a model for working on the plan with a defined frame for the treatment. There is a specific task in mind with a therapist, who is outside their relationship, functions as a "third" (Morgan, 2001), and tries to help them accomplish this goal. The parenting plan is used, both consciously and unconsciously, as a real and symbolic object, to help make individual and couple developmental changes. The conscious task is to create a document that can serve as a point of reference about the shared parenting agreements for the couple. Unconsciously, the parenting plan serves symbolically as a type of transitional object that facilitates a developmental process.

## The parenting plan as a transitional object

The parenting plan may be understood in terms of Winnicott's theory of transitional objects and transitional phenomena. According to Winnicott, the transitional object is "the first not-me possession," and enables the infant to find comfort in an external object, when its primary needs are not met. This process manifests when the "good enough mother" allows the impingement of reality to gradually emerge, and the infant finds comfort in an external object, as he or she learns to tolerate disappointment and frustration. The object serves as a container for internalised experiences, represents movement from fantasy to reality, and facilitates the emergence of the baby as separate from their caretaker. Illusion provides the domain for the transitional phenomena, the bridge between the subjective and the objective worlds. As an illusion, the transitional object represents the infant's transition from a state of being merged with the mother to a state of being in relation to the mother, as something outside and separate that allows for the acceptance of difference (Winnicott, 1953).

If transitional objects can be conceived as any object that conveys security to an individual in the absence of the source of that security, then transitional objects can be viewed as developmental facilitators (Garber, 2019). As the child moves towards physical and emotional independence, transitional objects serve different psychological functions. In this way, transitional objects can extend beyond childhood, serve as a bridge between any developmental stage, and still carry the illusion of the previous stage (Murray, 1974). According to Winnicott, no human being is ever free of the pressure of understanding their inner and outer reality, and everyone must cope with what he termed "intermediate areas of experience" or "transitional phenomena" (Winnicott, 1953).

This view of transitional phenomena is useful in understanding the intrapsychic and interpersonal dynamics of high-conflict couples in multiple dimensions. First, as they are forced to face the reality of their separation and divorce, the partners need to cope with their own internal anxieties about these changes. Secondly, they must manage their overwhelming emotional experiences, as they interact with one another in the external world. Due to an incapacity to tolerate these intrapsychic and interpersonal transitions, they endlessly battle in order to stay psychically together.

Co-parent therapy, and the parenting plan, can provide a secure container for the couple struggling with anxieties about psychic separateness during these transitions. The "good enough therapist," like the "good enough mother," provides a safe enough environment for the couple to better cope with their deep feelings of disappointment and loss. The creation of the plan gives them a new form of relating that allows them to be more psychically separate, while relating as a co-parent couple. Just as the transitional object for a child symbolises the mother and the breast, but it is *not* the breast or the mother, the parenting plan can symbolise an in-between, transitional space: the couple is no longer a marital couple and is now a more separate, independent co-parent couple (Murray, 1974).

According to Winnicott (1953), in normal development, the transitional object becomes gradually decathected, and there is a weakening, or a diffusion, of the emotional association to the transitional object. In accordance with Winnicott's theory, the parenting plan can facilitate development and become decathected. Although some couples will rely on the parenting plan throughout the years of their shared parenting, others may gradually give it up. It can function like a transitional object and lose its significance over time. Just like the child's blanket or teddy bear, the parenting plan does not need to be forgotten or mourned, but rather, it is no longer needed in the same way and its function has been transformed (Murray, 1974). When the co-parent therapy and the parenting plan have been internalised, the couple will become more able to relate as a co-parent couple.

However, the therapist can never fully know how the plan is perceived or used once the co-parenting therapy has ended. Even when co-parent therapy is effective, at times of regression, under the stress of external pressures, or when circumstances change, the co-parent couple may return to co-parent therapy seeking help with modifying their dynamics and shoring up parts of their parenting plan. This is an opportunity to continue to work with unresolved issues that may be interfering with the ability of the co-parent couple to parent their children.

### Clinical vignettes

**Nancy and Roger**, a divorced couple, were in a bitter legal battle over their custody arrangement. Nancy had been given temporary custody over Donald, their 12-year-old son, after she accused Roger of verbally abusing Donald. The court sent the couple to co-parent therapy to facilitate a therapeutic reconciliation between father and son, and for the parents to develop a parenting plan as Roger was regaining equal parenting time. During the reconciliation phase of the work, Nancy and Roger were surprisingly able to work together in helping their son manage his feelings of sadness and anger about his parents' divorce. Donald was furious with his mother who was in a new relationship, confirming for Donald that his parents' marriage was over. He was angry and acting out his anger in both parents' homes. In my assessment, Nancy tried to manage Donald's anger by being overly permissive of Donald's abusive behaviour towards her. Roger tried to manage Donald's anger by retaliation and punishment. Neither of these interventions seemed to be helpful to Donald.

I met with Donald alone, Donald with each parent, and with the three of them together. During the family work, Donald, who was quite articulate, was able to talk about his sadness and cry about his parent's divorce. He said that he felt like he no longer had a home and that his life, as he knew it, had vanished. In my office, the parents were able to listen to Donald's feelings and share his grief. They spoke about their own sadness about the loss of the family unit, and each of their culpability for the difficulties in their relationship with Donald. Donald seemed to calm down in response to his parents' empathy and attunement, and this translated to better behaviour at home.

In retrospect, my expectations of Nancy and Roger, following the success of the family work, were unrealistically high when we moved into the work on the parenting plan. Roger, having regained his parenting time with Donald, seemed to feel vindicated and victorious. He refused to communicate in a reliable way with me, and only sporadically attended appointments. I began to wonder if Roger had been previously manipulating me and Nancy, in order to regain his parenting time. Nancy was endlessly complaining about Roger's temper, his parenting, and his constant denigration of her. Roger was furious with Nancy, would barely speak to her, and complained about her disorganisation and lax parenting. I wondered if the previous parental alignment achieved had, paradoxically, caused profound anxiety and was replaced with a resumption of defensive splitting.

The split was also manifested in the transference. Roger was blatantly contemptuous of me and my role, and Nancy saw me as helpfully aligned with her. In my view, the parents were in a projective gridlock whereby Nancy was projecting her feelings about being an inadequate parent onto Roger, and in return he resentfully tried to put the bad parenting onto her. Despite my attempts to understand the couple and avoid joining in the enactment, I was worried that my own countertransference feelings might emerge in a dysregulated way. I felt aversive to Roger's constant denigration of me, his rage, and sarcasm. I felt impatient with Nancy's passivity, her inability to acknowledge her role in the problems, and her difficulties with parenting. Despite my attempts to facilitate their communication, respond to each of their emotional pain, and point out their projections (to each other and to me), I felt pressure to align with one of them at the expense of the other. My attempts to address their defences, as a way of shifting away from underlying feelings of loss, were met with steadfast defiance and professional threats against me. My countertransference feelings escalated to fears of annihilation and the impulse to terminate the therapy. I understood these feelings as emblematic of their own malevolent and persecutory experience, but it was difficult to tolerate nonetheless. Eventually, my refusal to collude with either of them led to their banding against me. They both accused me of being an incompetent, unprofessional therapist and left the treatment. Ironically, despite this ending, I believe they were able to utilise some version of the parenting plan that we had developed together. However, they continued to be a highly conflictual and fused couple, but now, united in a battle against me.

> The internal world of this couple was dominated by helplessness, fear, and destructive rage. This created significant distortions in their thought processes, leading to deeply damaging consequences for them and their child. This case demonstrates that, despite all of our skills, creativity, and attempts to understand the profound underlying psychopathology often present in high-conflict couples, for some, the level of pathology is just too complex to disentangle the deep rages and wounds necessary to become a co-parent couple.
>
> (Donner, 2006)

**Carol and Ron** came to see me when their children were thirteen and ten years old. We worked together weekly for four years. Before coming to my office, they had been embroiled in court battles, accomplishing nothing more than making a parenting time schedule. The children were on a week on/week off schedule, and the parents would not permit them to have any contact with either parent during the other parent's time.

The parents accused each other as being responsible for the breakup of the marriage, and they were rigidly implanted in polarised positions. They were caught in a repetitive cycle of blame, and were punishing each other by denying the other access to the children. Their behaviour in my office was volatile. They refused to look at each other, would only speak directly to me, and shouted at each other throughout many of the sessions. I was challenged to contain my countertransference feelings of frustration and hopelessness, and tried to refrain from enacting this by joining in their control struggles.

Since neither parent could support their children interacting with the other parent, a major goal of the co-parent therapy was to help them understand how to tolerate their children having relationships with both of them. Their gridlocked interactions were difficult for me to dislodge, prompting me to intervene in several ways. I tried to actively contain them, by telling them to stop yelling at one another. At other times, I would give advice regarding the importance of the children having a relationship with each parent. I would interpret the splitting, and the deeper destructive, controlling dynamics. For example, I suggested the fights over the children served to ward off the feelings of loss regarding the marriage and the family.

We started each session with an "agenda" of general parenting issues. We used the development of the parenting plan as an external organising structure to help them learn, recognise, and accept their differences in their evolving co-parent relationship. The clinical aims were to help them tolerate their psychological separateness, modify the persecutory quality of the relationship, and help them co-parent cooperatively. This allowed them access to deeper feelings of disappointment and loss. In the transference, they sometimes experienced me as a benevolent judge, and at other times, as a good mother. However, inevitably I became the focus of their anger, and they experienced me as unhelpful and deficient. They often resorted to splitting, whereby they each felt persecuted by me, and accused me of aligning with the other parent.

Over time, this couple's feelings gradually became modified in intensity and more regulated. They were able to rely on me, the co-parent therapy, and the parenting plan, and better function as a co-parent couple to the benefit of their children. After the end of the treatment, and when one of their children was preparing to go to college, Carol requested that I read her son's college essay. He had poignantly written about himself as a child who felt he had to be one son in his mother's house, and a different son in his father's house. I understood this as an expression of the splitting in the family, and of his difficulty having access to good and bad feelings for both parents. For much of his childhood, he felt there were two separate parts of him: he couldn't feel love for his father in his mother's house; nor love for his mother in his father's house. In the college essay, he wrote that he was now able to integrate these separate parts of himself, and see all that he was able to receive from his mother, and all that he was able to receive from his father. He felt that he had become one son with both his parents.

The formation of the parenting plan and psychoanalytic co-parent therapy helped this couple address the cycle of blaming and destructiveness that emanated from their inability to see each other as two separate entities. The treatment minimised their defensive splitting, modified their thinking and behaviour, helped them gain insight with regard to the defensive avoidance of their feelings of loss, and relate as a co-parent couple. As can be seen in this case, psychoanalytic co-parent therapy, along with the parenting plan, can function well as a developmental facilitator for both parents and children.

## Conclusion

The model put forth in this paper stems from my experience working with high-conflict separating and divorcing couples in California, in the United States. Approaches that primarily emphasise parenting and communication skills, without a more in-depth focus, are insufficient to address the complicated dynamics of high-conflict separating and divorcing couples. In contrast, viewing these couples through a psychoanalytic lens enables the therapist to help the partners become more psychologically separate, reduce their rage and destructive aggression, and allow access to their feelings of loss.

The co-parent therapy that I have described is applicable to working with a range of high-conflict couples, with greater or lesser psychological disturbance. However, in the most challenging cases, when the individuals in the couple are so fused by hate and bitter disappointment, and when they are unable to psychologically separate from one another, hatred drives the interactions, regardless of the impact on the children. When animosity becomes the motivating factor, conflict resolution is not possible (Demby, 2009). When the impulse to destroy the other parent is more important than working together for the benefit of their children, it is extremely difficult to unlock this type of dynamic. In these cases, couples generally do not remain in co-parent therapy and return to court for continued litigation.

Other high-conflict couples, despite their psychological difficulties, are able to derive benefit from psychoanalytically informed co-parent therapy. This approach offers containment for the intense dysregulated feelings, diminishes splitting and projection, facilitates psychological separation, examines irrational thinking, identifies hatred and destructiveness, and potentially modifies behaviour. A key component of this model rests on the creation of an individualised parenting plan, a document that functions on both a conscious and unconscious level. The parenting plan serves as a reference, a concrete document, that contains the couple's agreements about their shared parenting policies. It also functions on an unconscious, symbolic level, as a type of transitional object that facilitates development and creates new meaning for their dissolving relationship.

> It is in the space between inner and outer world, which is also the space between people--the transitional space--that intimate relationships and creativity occur.
>
> (Winnicott, 1953)

Borrowing from Winnicott, an environment that holds the couple well enough and allows for transitional space, enables personal development, and creative tendencies will evolve. This results in a continuity in the sense of self, an experience of the self that eventually results in autonomy (Winnicott, 1986). Similarly, a developmental shift towards separateness, achieved in co-parent therapy, is essential to the couple's ability to transition to a co-parent couple and find new, more cooperative ways of relating to one another. These changes are not only important for the couple – they will be internalised, communicated to the children, create less conflict, mitigate the enduring impact of the loss, and benefit the entire family.

## References

Bagnini, C. (2003). Containing anxiety with divorcing couples. In: Scharff, J. & Tsigounis, S.A. (eds.), *Self hatred in psychoanalysis: Detoxifying the persecutory object* (pp. 165–178). London: Routledge. 2003.

Clulow, C. (1990). Divorce as bereavement: Similarities and differences. *Family and Conciliation Courts Review*, 28(1): 19–22.

Colman, W. (1993). Marriage as a psychological container. In: Ruszczynski, S. (ed.), *Psychotherapy with couples: Theory and practice at the Tavistock Institute of Marital Studies* (pp. 70–96). London: Karnac.

Demby, S. (2009). Interparent hatred and Its impact on parenting: Assessment in forensic custody evaluations. *Psychoanalytic Inquiry*, 29(6): 477–490.

Donner, M. (2006). Tearing the child apart: The contribution of narcissism, envy, and perverse modes of thought to child custody wars. *Psychoanalytic Psychology*, 23(3): 542–553.

Ehrenberg, M., & Hunter, M. (1996). Shared parenting agreements after marital separation: The roles of empathy and narcissism. *Journal of Consulting and Clinical Psychology*, 64(4): 808–818.

Garber, B. (2019). For the love of fluffy: Respecting, protecting, and empowering transitional objects in the context of high conflict divorce. *Journal of Divorce & Remarriage*, 60(7): 552–565.

Johnston, J., & Campbell, L. (1988). *Impasses of divorce: The dynamics and resolutions of family conflict*. London: Macmillan.

Lasso, R. (2003). Divorce terminable and interminable: A psychoanalytic and interdisciplinary approach. *Journal of Applied Psychoanalytic Studies*, 5(3): 321–334.

Levite, Z., & Cohen, O. (2011). The tango of loving hate: Couple dynamics in high-conflict divorce. *Journal of Clinical Social Work*, 40, 46–55.

Morgan, M. (1995). The projective gridlock: A form of projective identification in couple relationships. In: Ruszczynski, S. & Fischer, J. (eds.), *Intrusiveness and intimacy in the couple* (pp. 33–48). London: Karnac.

Morgan, M. (2001). First contacts: The therapist's "couple state of mind" as a factor in the containment of couples seen for consultations. In: Grier, F. (ed.), *Brief encounters with couples* (pp. 17–32). London: Karmac.

Murray, M.E. (1974). The therapist as a transitional object. *American Journal of Psychoanalysis*, 34: 123–127.

Nathans, S., & Schaefer, M. (2017). *Couples on the couch: Psychoanalytic couple therapy and the Tavistock Model*. New York: Routledge.

Nyberg, V., & Hertzmann, L. (2019). Mentalization-based couple therapy. In A. Balfour, C. Clulow, & K. Thompson (eds.), *Engaging couples: new directions in therapeutic work with families* (pp. 130–143). London: Routledge.

Ruszczynski, S.P. (1992). Notes towards a psychoanalytic understanding of the couple relationship. *Psychoanalytic Psychotherapy*, 6(1): 33–48.

Ruszczynski, S.P. (1993). Thinking about working with couples. In: Ruszczynski, S. (ed.), *Psychotherapy with couples: Theory and practice at the Tavistock Institute of Marital Studies* (pp. 197–217). London: Karnac.

Scharff, K.E. (2004) Therapeutic supervision with families of high-conflict divorce. *International Journal of Applied Psychoanalytic Studies*, 1(3): 269–281.

Shmueli, A. (2005) On thinking of parents as adults in divorce and separation. *Sexual and Relationship Therapy*, 20(3): 349–357.

Shmueli, A. (2012). Working therapeutically with high conflict divorce. In: Balfour, A., Morgan, M., & Vincent, C. (eds.), *How couple relationships shape our world* (pp. 137–158). London: Karnac.

Vincent, C. (2001). Giving advice durinsg consultations: Unconscious enactment or thoughtful containment? In: Grier, F. (ed.), *Brief encounters with couples* (pp. 85–97). London: Karmac.

Winnicott, D.W. (1953). Transitional objects and transitional phenomena – a study of the first not-me possession. *International Journal of Psychoanalysis*, 34: 89–97.

Winnicott, D.W. (1986). *Home is where we start from: Essays by a psychoanalyst.* Winnicott, C., Shepard, R. & Davis, M. (eds.). New York: Norton.

# Chapter 18

# Discussion of "Co-parent therapy and the parenting plan as transitional phenomena"

## Working psychoanalytically with high-conflict separating and divorcing couples

*Avi Shmueli*

The central tenant of the chapter by Dana Iscoff is the use of the concrete tool, the parenting plan, which is used to engage a couple in a psychoanalytic process that enables them to develop and retain their role as parents while also divorced. As she states: "the parenting plan may serve as a transitional object for the couple, facilitating their psychological development, and aiding in their transition from a separating or divorcing couple to a co-parent couple." The parenting plan itself is defined in a very literal manner as "an individualised and detailed list of agreements, rules, and policies related to the parenting time schedule and shared parental responsibilities" (Iscoff, this volume, p. 231).

The challenge is formidable because, from a psychoanalytic perspective, a couple creates a projective system which may be colloquially referred to as the "couple dance." Each of the partners unconsciously uses the relationship as a forum within which to try to resolve past difficulties (Ruszczynski, 1993). Therefore, each uses projective identification to try and convey these difficulties, but they simultaneously need to defend against the psychic pain involved (Shmueli, 2012). This balance in the couple relationship, between a developmental wish and a defensive push-back, sets the scene for the future of the relationship and consequently the different types of divorce (Clulow & Vincent, 1987).

Separation and divorce are regarded as the second most stressful life events, only surpassed by the death of a child (Holmes & Rahe, 1967). These experiences are regarded as more stressful than being imprisoned, moving house, or getting married. The difficulties inherent to high-conflict couples are difficult to precisely define (Shmueli, 2012). Perhaps Iscoff's choice to focus on high-conflict couples

DOI: 10.4324/9781003265023-18

originated from the fact that this degree of conflict is likely to promote physical and concrete responses, rather than maintain a purely psychic nature of response. A parenting plan that is literal and concrete may therefore appeal to such couples.

This discussion will address three aspects of the work outlined by Iscoff, each of which are inherent and crucial to the task itself. These are (i) the provision of orientation for the couple, (ii) the provision of hope in the implicit assumption of development, and (iii) the protection of the child(ren) from the projections of the parents. I will also point out two aspects that may serve as contraindications to attempting to establish a parenting plan: the irretrievable loss of the "good" alongside the purpose of projective identification in the parental couple relationship; and the therapist's own capacity to maintain the required mental state in the clinical setting.

## The provision of orientation

No couple becomes involved with each other with a view to eventual separation. Indeed, it is difficult to imagine a relationship into which more is invested than the couple marital/co-habiting relationship. Consequently, separation and divorce are not only stressful but profoundly disorienting. In another paper, I described how the process of separation and divorce requires the couple to simultaneously function within three independent domains (Shmueli, 2012). Most easily identifiable is the *Environmental domain* which constitutes the management of very tangible and essentially conscious factors, such as finance, moves of home, changes of routine, and the legal process itself. Such changes require conscious attention at a level of detail that, prior to the divorce, may simply not have been necessary. It is a paradox that at the time a couple wishes to separate, they may also have to work together at a degree of detail previously unachieved.

Simultaneously, each of the individuals in the divorcing couple must address within themselves the experience of a loss that was not envisaged by either when the couple were first lovers. Each must mourn the loss of the relationship, even if the divorce has been longed for. This second domain has been called the *Preconscious Normative Domain*, borrowing Freud's term, in his topographical model of the mind (Freud, 1900). The term preconscious is used because the experience of loss has to be consciously acknowledged even if there is resistance to achieving this. The term normative is used because there is very little choice in having to experience divorce as a bereavement, even if individuals differ in how they process this loss. While different models of grief, such as Bowlby's four-stage model (Protest, Yearning, Despair, and Reorganisation) (Bowlby, 1980), or Kubler-Ross' (2008) five-stage model (Denial, Anger, Bargaining, Depression, Acceptance), may apply, but each and every divorcing individual will be faced with the normal necessity of grieving for the relationship.

The third domain that profoundly influences the passage through and management of the Environmental and Preconscious Normative Domains is the *Unconscious Idiopathic Domain*. This is the domain of an individual unconscious phantasy upon which one-half of the couple's projective cycle was based. Colloquially speaking, it is the domain in which the unique essence of each person and their individuality resides. The specificity of these phantasies is part and parcel of the individual's psychic functioning and therefore effectively dictates other functioning. They are the lens through which all else is viewed.

The disorientation and stress of divorce and separation thus emerge from the fact that change occurs in all three domains simultaneously, and for a potentially protracted period. Such is the impact that the individual's very sense of identity may be threatened, and hence the potential for entrenched conflict with the soon-to-be ex-partner will be increased. The role of the parenting plan may therefore be crucial at such times. In being a product of psychotherapeutic work, while also being both literal and specific, the parenting plan may provide a vital point of orientation for the couple. It potentially can encapsulate enough of these domains to allow each individual to feel represented and therefore able to collaborate.

## The provision of hope and development

While Winnicott considered transitional objects as an important part of development from the perspective of the child, it is not too difficult to suggest that the child itself functions as a representation of the parent's own past investment and future hopes. The divorce, and threatened loss of contact with children, can thus be experienced as a threat to the individual's own life and capacity to function. Under the influence of the phantasy of "psychic death," the child can very easily become the principal focus of the parent's projections. The child is thus no longer the separate product of the parent's union but is unconsciously treated as the representative of the parent for future life. Simultaneously, the consciously felt future for either or both the parents can appear bleak, and hence the prospect of entrenched conflict may serve to provide a lifeline for them, even though this might not appear to be the case.

The description of the parenting plan by Iscoff implicitly captures both the role of each parent in the child's past, and the ongoing involvement in the child's future. This is further emphasised by the fact that the plan is the creation of the couple in conjunction with the therapist. Crucially, the embodiment of this aspect of the plan allows for the ownership of the plan, rather than ownership of the child as a representation of the future. Thus, the specificity of the parenting plan, in addition to what it represents, can act as a transitional object for the parents and thus facilitate development. It can implicitly be a representation of hope for the individuals and their capacity to function in the future.

## The protection of children

It is difficult to over-estimate the investment made by each partner in the other, especially when the consciously spoken statements of each partner suggest an entirely different picture. However, it is in the link with the projective cycle that the origins of the eventual separation can be observed. Elsewhere I have suggested that the projective cycle be likened to the shell of an egg in its being able to withstand enormous pressures when intact, and yet being highly fragile when cracked (Shmueli, 2019). The crack itself may occur from within due to developments within the egg or may occur from without in the form of an external trauma. So it is for the divorcing couple, with the separation triggered by the psychological development of either or both the partners, and from without as a consequence of an event that the projective cycle cannot manage.

This "fracture" in the container implies that projections between the couple cannot ordinarily be expected to either be withdrawn or cease. More likely, they find another home, namely the children and the lawyers. This is very different to the children being thought about. The child itself, by virtue of being dependent upon the parents, is highly vulnerable to the projections of the parents. Target et al. (2017)

completed a qualitative study exploring the experience of contact arrangements for high-conflict divorced couples. A thematic analysis of responses to a semi structured interview yielded three prominent themes. Firstly, "dealing with contact evokes extreme states of mind"; secondly. the child is "everywhere and nowhere" in the parents' narrative; and thirdly, "the hardest thing about contact is dealing with my ex-partner." Taken as a group, these themes strongly suggest that these parents cannot conceptualise the child as a separate independent entity requiring care, but only see the child as an extension of themselves, as a collection of diverted projections. Thus arises the experience of many clinicians sitting with parents arguing over what their child ate the previous evening, each convinced of the correctness of their view.

Iscoff's use of the parenting plan as a tool is innovative because it potentially establishes an alternative forum, an alternative shell, within which the parent's projections may be housed. More importantly, it potentially maintains the child as conceptually separate from the parent and, as such, serves to protect the child from the extremes of the parents' projections.

## The case illustration of Carol and Ron

Iscoff's description of Carol and Ron is very interesting both in its modesty and in the way it captures many of the points discussed above. Limitations of space preclude an extended discussion, but several points are worthy of mention. The parents presented the paradox of each having to orient themselves through the denial of the reality of the other, a split that could not be maintained over time given their children's development but was at times desperately clung to and echoed in their son's essay. Interestingly, the thinking behind Iscoff's therapeutic actions is not expanded upon in her paper, but it does illustrate many of the dilemma's faced by therapists working in the field of divorce and separation.

The fact that the work with Carol and Ron spanned four years illustrates the very different pace of the legal and psychological processes: in separation and divorce, the psychological processes take much longer than the legal ones. At the same time, for this couple, the use of an agenda at the beginning of sessions seemed to represent the presence of hope and development. This included developments for each of the parents in mourning their respective losses, which of course did not feel like development in the moment but are very much part of this process.

Throughout, and implicit in Iscoff's work, observation and work in the transference prevailed, and this reflects the psychoanalytic orientation of the model she employs. This served as part of the experience of developing the parenting plan and thus enabled the development of their children's identity as the product of both parents.

Finally, the case of Carol and Ron illustrates the incompleteness and imperfection inherent to working with divorcing couples, Carol conveyed the developments that had occurred principally through sending Iscoff the essay, rather than being able to describe it directly with the ex-husband in the room. Therapists working in this field learn to understand the evidence of implicit change and development, rather than requiring explicit statements.

## Contraindications to the use of a parenting plan

Winnicott's concept of transitional phenomena (Winnicott, 1975) relies on the objects being positively cathected and therefore felt as "good." The child's doll successfully functions as a transitional object only because it predominantly represents the positively cathected experiences with the parents. The implication of this for the parenting plan are threefold.

Firstly, the therapist's capacity to maintain the distinction between the patient's internal world, which operates according to very different rules, and the external world is crucial (Parsons, 2007). While this capacity is often taken for granted in being a psychotherapist, it is especially important when working in the field of divorce and separation, given the intensity of the transference–countertransference experiences generated. This capacity, and the view of each individual as lying on a developmental trajectory, is necessary for understanding the patient's experience and is essential for providing hope. This does not mean that the therapist forsakes the "couple state of mind" (Morgan, 2019). The central feature of separating couples, and particularly high-conflict couples, is the presence of the fracture in the couple projective system. The therapist is required to be able to understand the nature of the development that has occurred while simultaneously understanding the fracture. In other words, the therapist needs to be able to observe the fate of the projections and be able to see both individuals as linked developing individuals, rather than as part of a couple. A lack of robustness on the part of the therapist in this regard means that the evocation of an experience of psychic death will dominate the therapeutic work and will likely be reinforced by the concrete and external nature of the divorce and separation. This scenario will condemn the parenting plan to failure.

Secondly, and implicitly as part of considering transitional phenomena, it is crucial that each of the partners in the couple can or can be helped to identify the "good," positively cathected aspects of themselves, these aspects were undoubtedly present at the beginning of the relationship but may not be so readily available in the process of divorce. Without these aspects being held in mind or at least present in the therapist's mind, it seems unlikely that the parenting plan could evolve to become the transitional object that is hoped for.

Thirdly, any clinician familiar with couple psychotherapy would testify to the complexity and multiply layered nature of every couple relationship. It is this very fact that makes the couple relationship such a forum for psychological development. However, as mentioned previously, the projective cycle for each couple arrives with a tension between the push for development and the need for defence. A predominance of defence over development highlights the differing purposes of the projective identification between the partners. While ordinary relating through projective identification is considered to have a communicative intent, it may conversely be dominated by an evacuative intent. In these cases, the denial and projection results in the partners locating these split off aspects of the self in their partner. The vehemence of such evacuations can squash any possibility of thinking that the reality may be different and is maintained against all efforts to understand it. Under such circumstances, separating will be difficult because the process requires some degree of a re-introjection of what was initially projected. The pressure will be on the parenting plan to incorporate the projective system as is, which will potentially be a repetition of the situation which brought the couple to divorcing. In my opinion, when the therapist can identify the primary functioning in the projective cycle as being evacuative, the use of such a tool as the parenting plan is ill advised.

Iscoff's example of Nancy and Roger usefully illustrates some of these points. From the description available, the shared phantasy for the couple lay in the phantasy that aggression could only be destructive. Therefore, the ongoing battle between them took the form of mutual recrimination as to which of then was being crueller. The court itself was drawn into the "fight" in using its authority to force the couple to attend therapy and unwittingly, in my opinion, enacted the very dynamic between the couple. Throughout this, the couple's son was the mouthpiece for distress. Iscoff's description of the work conveys the intense pressure she came under, and the robustness required to maintain the work with this couple. It is clear to see how the couple's use of the child in the service of their difficulties was lessened because of the therapeutic work, and he undoubtedly benefitted from this. This was accompanied by an increase in the intensity of the transference in which Iscoff became the devalued, contemptible, and hated object that had been part of the couple's projective system. Her capacity to work with this is to her credit, but as she acknowledges, the picture that emerges is of a couple who were never able to digest this aspect and consequently perpetually evacuated this to each other in the projective cycle. There was little "good" that was readily available to them. Any re-introjection required for development would have been experienced by each of them as acceptance of their own overall and fundamental "badness," and this had to be resisted at all costs. While the work therefore provided needed respite for their son, under these circumstances, it is difficult to imagine that a parenting plan had any hope of success.

## Final comment

The concept of the parenting plan as a transitional phenomenon and a transitional object is undoubtedly both interesting and clinically useful. In my view, it is cutting-edge because psychoanalysis does not usually employ concrete and prospective techniques. It is important to recognise that, in Iscoff's conceptualization, the parenting plan is the outcome of the psychotherapeutic work, rather than the ultimate aim of the work. The development of a parenting plan represents the work done, rather than being a substitute for it, and this is illustrated by Iscoff's useful and honest depiction of the two cases reported.

As a product of therapeutic work, the parenting plan has further potential as an outcome measure for such applied work. For example, it would be extremely interesting to follow up with a case such as Carol and Ron. It would be useful to understand how well they were able to adhere to the parenting plan and learn if they were able to continue to develop it (and themselves) as their children grew up. As such, the parenting plan can become even more the internal "child" of the couple's therapeutic work and will be less related to the external child, whom it was initially designed to protect.

# References

Bowlby, J. (1980) *Attachment and loss III: Loss, sadness and depression*. London: Hogarth Press.

Clulow, C., & Vincent, C. (1987) *In the child's best interests: Divorce court welfare and the search for a settlement*. London: Tavistock.

Freud, S. (1900) *The interpretation of dreams*. Standard Edition Vol IV. New York: Vintage.

Holmes, T., & Rahe, R. (1967) The social readjustment rating scale. *Journal of Psychosomatic Research*, *11*(2): 213–218.

Kubler-Ross, E. (2008) *Death and dying*. London: Routledge.

Morgan, M. (2019). *A couple state of mind: Psychoanalysis of couples and the Tavistock relationships model*. London: Routledge.

Parsons, M. (2007). Raiding the inarticulate: The internal analytic setting and listening beyond countertransference. *International Journal of Psychoanalysis*, *88*(6): 1441–1456. doi: 10.1516/T564-G13J-400H-2W23

Ruszczynski, S. (1993) *Psychotherapy with couples: Theory and practice at the Tavistock Institute of Marital Studies*. London: Karnac.

Shmueli, A. (2012). Working therapeutically with high conflict divorce. In: A. Balfour, M. Morgan, & C. Vincent (Eds.), *How couple relationships shape our world: Clinical practice, research, and policy perspectives* (pp. 137–158). London: Karnac.

Shmueli, A. (2019). Working with the fractured container. In: A. Balfour, C. Clulow, & K. Thompson (Eds.), *Engaging couples: New directions in therapeutic work with families* (pp. 169–182). London: Routledge.

Target, M., Hertzmann, L., Midgley, N., Casey, P., & Lassria, D. (2017). Parents' experience of child contact within entrenched conflict families following separation and divorce: A qualitative study. *Psychoanalytic Psychotherapy*, *31*(2), 218–246.

Winnicott, D.W. (1975).*Through paediatrics to psycho-analysis*. London: Karnac.

# Index

real objects (role) 10; receptive
unconscious 7; repetition 13;
technique 10–11; use of objects
16–17
Bollas, C. (works): *Meaning and
Melancholia* (2018) 6; *Mystery
of Things* (1999) 18; *Shadow of
Object* (1987) 6
Boston Change Process Study
Group 194
Bowlby, John 85, 143; four-stage
model of grief 244
British Independent Tradition 1, 6
Britton, Ron xii, 76, 86, 211, 221;
on Father Christmas 120; post-
Kleinian 2; unconscious facts 120

caregivers and caregiving 14, 85,
129, 157
castration anxieties 106, 177,
185–186
central ego (Fairbairn) 143, 148,
150–151
Chagall, Marc 185
Chicago xxiv, 198, 212
childhood 89, 103–107, 146, 157,
202–203, 226; son of divorced
parents 238
children: high-conflict couples
226–227, 229, 243–246, 249;
protection (divorcing parents)
245–246
Clarke, Graham 144
claustro-agoraphobic narrative xiv,
85, 87–88
claustrophobic anxieties 66
clinical imagination 24–25;
definition 1, 24
Clulow, C. xviii, 85
Cohen, J. 78–79
collaborative empathetic
interpretation (Leone) 205,
207, 223
Colman, Warren 1–2, 85, 98; gesture
11–12
coming out 123–124, 135–138, 146
communication xiv, 5–6, 11, 13, 24,
30–31, 230, 236, 238; nonverbal
28; problems 169–170, 173

compliance 14, 28–29
connectedness 196, 206, 213
contempt 15, 105, 163, 193, 235, 249
control system versus need system
(Fairbairn) 148
Controversial Discussions
(Klein versus Anna Freud,
1942–1944) 143
Cooke, Rachel xvi, xviii, 211–223;
biographical note xxii
co-parent therapy xvi, 225–250
"core complex" theory: absence of
sex from couple relationships xiv,
84–110; exclusion of father 103
countertransference 49, 113, 122,
126–127, 151–154, 230, 235–236,
247; experience 91, 93, 95–97, 99;
reaction xv, 34
couple 23; capacity for passion
40–41; dance 242; "fantastically
complicated system" 20–21;
feeling "real" 53–55; identity
168, 185; link theory 166–188;
narcissistic foundation 170–171;
need for representation 170–171;
origin as illusion 171–173; point
of breakdown 169; traumatised
(work of psychoanalysts) 30; as
use of a plural 167–169
couple fit (Balint and Pincus)
144, 153
couple psychoanalytic theory 81
couple psychotherapy 1, 72–73, 228;
application of self psychology
xvi, 190–223; constant dialectic
162; mood and atmosphere 28;
new branch of psychoanalytic
therapy 150
couple relationships 183, 248;
absence of sex ("core complex"
lens) xiv, 84–110; foundational
myth 172–173, 184–185; loss and
disillusionment 78–80; stifling of
creativity 27
couple's superego 117, 120–121
couple state of mind 219, 221, 247;
explanation 230
couple therapists, role 164
COVID-19 pandemic xxii, 78–79

Simon, Paul 58
single parent families 62, 141
social environment xv, 167
social structure xv, 180, 183–184
socio-cultural environment 117, 132–133, 137, 139
splitting xvi, 64, 143, 162–163
spontaneous gesture 11, 14, 22
Steiner, John xii, 211
Stein, R. 127
Stevenson, Robert Louis 38
Stolorow, R. 191
stress 223; divorce 243–244
superego xv, 10, 39, 69, 103, 114, 117–121, 124; development 68, 133; individual versus cultural 117–118
Sutherland, J.D. 144–145, 148
systems, open and closed 151–152

tantrums 26
Target, M. 129, 134, 193, 214, 245–246
Tavistock Centre for Couple Relationships (London) xii
Tavistock Clinic 142, 150
Tavistock model xii, xv, xvi, xvii, 20, 47, 211, 214–216; technical considerations 219–223
Tavistock Relationships xii, xviii, xxiv–xxvi, 1
technique 10–11, 27
teenage man 66, 70–71, 80
Temperley, J. 76
therapist and client, selfobject bond 194–195
therapists 120, 122–124; battle against internalised homophobia 119–120; connectedness 196; clash with clients 234–236; function as "third" 232; "homophobic other" 125–127, 137; optimal responsiveness (Bacal) 196; paralysis 126–127; role 115; sense of paralysis xiv, 113; theory and practice 153–154; unconscious biases xv
third 63, 76, 86, 97, 99, 102, 105, 114–116, 173, 223, 232

third position (Britton) 86, 99, 105, 114–116, 127
trailing edge (problematic behaviour) 193–194, 206–207, 221
transference 156, 212, 230, 235, 237, 247, 249; repetition 219, 223
transitional objects (Winnicott) 51, 53, 242, 247, 249; parenting plan 232–234
transitional phenomena 51, 53, 248–249
transitional space 28–29
trauma 30, 61, 71, 82, 104, 145–147, 153, 185, 194, 205, 226, 245; Bollas's theory 29
traumatic confusion 59
triangular space 2, 115
triangulated emotional experience 113
triangulated relationships 103, 109
triangulation 107–108; rivalrous 64–65, 76; split-object 64–66, 70, 76
triggered states 30
trust 59, 75, 82, 88
two-person relationships 96–97, 103

unconscious xv, 15–16, 18, 27, 29, 135–138 *passim*, 144, 148, 150, 157–158, 211, 215; anxieties 60–61; beliefs 114, 120–121, 124; idiopathic domain 244; innate creativity 10–11; phantasy 1–2, 57, 89, 97–98, 113, 118, 167, 211, 244
United Kingdom 141, 150
United States 141, 180, 225; legal system (high-conflict separation and divorce) 227–228
unmetabolised loss 75, 77
unthought knowns 8, 10–11, 29

visual art xiii
vitalizing presence 55
vital sparks 50–51
vital spark (Winnicott) 50
Vorchheimer, Monica xix, 79; biographical note xxvii; link theory xv–xvi, 166–188
vulnerability 151

For Product Safety Concerns and Information please contact our EU
representative  GPSR@taylorandfrancis.com
Taylor & Francis Verlag GmbH, Kaufingerstraße 24, 80331 München, Germany

www.ingramcontent.com/pod-product-compliance
Lightning Source LLC
Chambersburg PA
CBHW052121230326
41598CB00080B/3937

9 78 1 0 3 2 2 0 7 4 5 2